Therapeutic Uses and Efficacy of Botulinum Toxin in Orofacial Medicine: From the Standpoint of Dental Professionals

Therapeutic Uses and Efficacy of Botulinum Toxin in Orofacial Medicine: From the Standpoint of Dental Professionals

Editors

Kazuya Yoshida
Merete Bakke

MDPI

Basel • Beijing • Wuhan • Barcelona • Belgrade • Novi Sad • Cluj • Manchester

Editors

Kazuya Yoshida
Kyoto Medical Center
Kyoto
Japan

Merete Bakke
University of Copenhagen
Copenhagen
Denmark

Editorial Office
MDPI AG
Grosspeteranlage 5
4052 Basel, Switzerland

This is a reprint of articles from the Special Issue published online in the open access journal *Toxins* (ISSN 2072-6651) (available at: https://www.mdpi.com/journal/toxins/special_issues/Botulinum_Toxin_Orofacial_Medicine).

For citation purposes, cite each article independently as indicated on the article page online and as indicated below:

Lastname, A.A.; Lastname, B.B. Article Title. *Journal Name* **Year**, *Volume Number*, Page Range.

ISBN 978-3-7258-2093-1 (Hbk)
ISBN 978-3-7258-2094-8 (PDF)
doi.org/10.3390/books978-3-7258-2094-8

Cover image courtesy of Kazuya Yoshida

Contents

About the Editors

Kazuya Yoshida

Kazuya Yoshida is the Head of the Department of Oral and Maxillofacial Surgery at the National Hospital Organization, Kyoto Medical Center, Kyoto, Japan. He graduated from Osaka Dental University, Osaka, Japan, in 1988 and was awarded a PhD, Doctor of Dentistry (Osaka Dental University), in 1992. He worked at the Free University of Berlin, Berlin, Germany, from 1992 to 1994. He worked at Kyoto University from 1994 to 2007, was awarded a PhD, Doctor of Medical Science (Kyoto University), in 2001, and from 2007 to present, he has worked at Kyoto Medical Center. His major research interests are clinical and neurophysiological research of movement disorders in the stomatognathic system, sleep apnea syndrome, and temporomandibular disorders. He applies a comprehensive range of treatments, including medication, oral appliance therapy, injection of botulinum toxin (Botox), and surgery (coronoidotomy), for involuntary movements in the orofacial region.

Merete Bakke

Merete Bakke DDS, PhD, Dr. Odont. and Swedish dental specialist (specialisttandläkare) is a Full Professor and Head of Clinical Oral Physiology at the Department of Odontology, Faculty of Health and Medical Sciences, University of Copenhagen, Denmark. Her major research area is temporomandibular function and disorders and associated orofacial pain. She has also worked at the Danish Headache Center, Rigshospitalet, and has collaborated on oromandibular dystonia with the Department of Neurology, Bispebjerg and Frederiksberg Hospitals, Bispebjerg, Copenhagen, Denmark.

Preface

The following Special Issue covers a wide range of topics, including neurological conditions such as oromandibular dystonia, pain-related disorders such as myofascial pain, primary headache, trigeminal or post-herpetic neuralgia, diseases of the temporomandibular joint such as temporomandibular joint disorder and bruxism, sialorrhea, and also cosmetic applications. The approved indications for botulinum toxin injections for each condition may vary between countries. To be officially approved for a certain indication, evidence from well-designed, randomized, controlled trials with larger sample sizes and longer follow-up periods is essential. To facilitate the use of botulinum toxin widely and routinely by general practitioners a guideline for safe and effective treatment must be established. In addition, differential diagnosis is important for neurological diseases, and collaboration between neurological and dental experts is advisable. Since dental professionals are specialists in the stomatognathic system, they may have the skills to diagnose and provide more accurate injections to target the muscles of interest in the oral region than medical professionals. Effective and safe botulinum toxin therapy requires a multidisciplinary team approach. We hope that botulinum therapy will become effective and safe for the treatment of various oral diseases more widely and that it will enable the treatment of many patients.

Kazuya Yoshida and Merete Bakke
Editors

toxins MDPI

Editorial

Therapeutic Uses and Efficacy of Botulinum Toxin in Orofacial Medicine: A Dental Perspective

Kazuya Yoshida [1,*] and Merete Bakke [2]

1 Department of Oral and Maxillofacial Surgery, National Hospital Organization, Kyoto Medical Center, 1-1 Mukaihata-cho, Fukakusa, Fushimi-ku, Kyoto 612-8555, Japan
2 Clinical Oral Physiology, Department of Odontology, Faculty of Health and Medical Sciences, University of Copenhagen, DK-2200 Copenhagen, Denmark; mbak@sund.ku.dk
* Correspondence: yoshida.kazuya.ut@mail.hosp.go.jp or omdystonia@gmail.com

Citation: Yoshida, K.; Bakke, M. Therapeutic Uses and Efficacy of Botulinum Toxin in Orofacial Medicine: A Dental Perspective. *Toxins* **2024**, *16*, 220. https://doi.org/10.3390/toxins16050220

Received: 28 March 2024
Accepted: 26 April 2024
Published: 10 May 2024

Botulinum neurotoxin (BoNT) is the exotoxin of *Clostridium botulinum*, a Gram-positive, spore-forming bacterium. Kerner was the first to describe botulism [1] and Van Ermengem isolated the microorganism *Bacillus Botulinus* [2] but it was not until 1979 that Scott was able to make the first use of BoNT therapeutically for strabismus via injection to the extraocular muscles [3]. The clinical applications of BoNT have since dramatically expanded to treat ophthalmic, neurological, gastrointestinal, urological, orthopedic, dermatological, dental, secretory, painful, and other diseases [4,5]. Moreover, applications to the orofacial region have gained particular attention [6], targeting disorders such as oromandibular dystonia (OMD), hemifacial spasm, facial synkinesis, orolingual dyskinesia, functional dystonia, hemimasticatory spasms, trigeminal neuralgia, orofacial pain, temporomandibular disorders, temporomandibular joint dislocation, bruxism, palatal tremor, hypersalivation, spasmodic dysphonia, essential voice tremor, first-bite syndrome, and Frey syndrome [6]. In most cases the temporal and the masseter muscles are injected bilaterally as standard; however, treatment effects may be hampered as dystonia, spasms, and dyskinesia with involuntary jaw and tongue movements may be misdiagnosed due to the complexity of muscle activity and the involvement of several small muscles [7].

This Special Issue is focused on the use of BoNT in the orofacial region, from a dental perspective. Five papers reported on pain-related disorders, with three of these focusing on myofascial pain [Contributions 1–3], one on trigeminal or post-herpetic neuralgia [Contribution 4], and one on primary headache [Contribution 5]. Another four papers focused on OMD or neurological conditions [Contributions 6–8], and we also have a narrative review on the cosmetic applications of BoNT [Contribution 9].

BoNT alleviates muscle tension and pain, which is why the masticatory muscle pain associated with temporomandibular disorders or bruxism seems to be the area of greatest interest among dentists and oral surgeons [8]. De la Torre Canales et al. [Contribution 1] conducted a randomized controlled trial on BoNT-A and its effects on mandibular range of motion (pain-free, maximum unassisted and assisted mouth opening, and right and left lateral mandibular movements) and muscle tenderness in 80 patients with persistent myofascial pain. The patients were randomly divided into four groups (n = 20): three BoNT-A groups with different doses and a saline solution control group. The examination was performed blindly and according to the RDC/TMD classification [9]. After 28 and 180 days of treatment, compared with the control group palpation pain over the masseter and temporalis muscles were significantly reduced in all three BoNT-A groups regardless of dose. They concluded that BoNT-A improved mandibular range of motion and muscle tenderness in patients with persistent myofascial pain and that the effect was dosage independent. De la Torre Canales et al. [Contribution 2] also assessed the long-term effects of BoNT-A for 72 months in terms of subjective pain (VAS), pain sensibility (PPT), and muscle thickness (ultrasonography) in 14 patients with the same malady. They concluded that a single injection of BoNT-A provided long-term pain reduction in patients with persistent myofascial pain, and a reversibility of the negative effect on masticatory muscle thickness. Sitnikova et al. [Contribution 3] conducted a randomized clinical trial of BoNT injection in 57 patients with myalgia, myofascial pain, or headache attributable according to the Diagnostic Criteria for Temporomandibular Disorders (DC/TMD) and considered the degree and duration of the impairment of muscle performance after BoNT injection. The patients were randomly divided into two groups: one of which received BoNT-A first ($n = 28$) while the other received saline first ($n = 29$), with a cross-over timetabled in week 16, and a total follow-up period of 32 weeks. In total, 50 units were used in each patient with 2/3 bilaterally in the masseter and 1/3 in the temporalis. A significant reduction in electromyographic activity was observed up to week 18 ($p \leq 0.001$), with full recovery at week 33. A significant reduction in the maximum bite force was observed up to week 11 ($p \leq 0.005$), with full recovery at week 25. They conclude that muscle function recovery occurred within 33 weeks after BoNT-A, and thus considered that to be the period after which reinjections would be safe. The management of neuropathic pain is also challenging, and patients with the condition are often under the care of a dentist or an oral surgeon. Val et al. [Contribution 4] provided a systematic review regarding the clinical application of BoNT in managing neuropathic pain in the orofacial region, in which they analyzed five randomized clinical trials on classical trigeminal neuralgia, and one trial on post-herpetic neuralgia. The review concluded that the evidence supports the efficacy of BoNT injections for orofacial neuropathic pain management and the authors suggested that study protocols should be improved by considering patient selection, phenotyping, injection techniques, dosing, intervals between doses, etc. Moreover, an increased homogeneity among the research protocols is required to provide a protocol for the tailored use of BoNT for different orofacial neuropathic pain conditions.

Primary headaches, otherwise termed idiopathic headaches, are a large group of diseases, the etiology of the primary headache is unclear, and it is not a symptom of another known disease. The most common of these are migraines, tension-type headaches, and cluster headaches. Kępczyńska and Domitrz conducted a narrative review on the use of BoNT in chronic migraine and other primary headaches [Contribution 5], finding that BoNT is effective in pain control through its interaction with the soluble NSF attachment protein receptor complex, which inhibits the release of neurotransmitters, such as glutamate, substance P, and calcitonin gene-related peptide. BoNT-A is effective not only in reducing headache frequency and pain intensity, but also in improving other parameters including sufferers' quality of life. They emphasize that many patients with these headaches seek dental care because orofacial pain is a common symptom; hence, an orofacial pain specialist should know about the diagnostic criteria for various types of headaches. Likewise, headache physicians should be aware of the semiologic aspects of orofacial pain.

Involuntary movements, such as dystonia, were the main target diseases when BoNT was first applied clinically [4,5]. OMD is a focal dystonia involving the masticatory, lingual, and/or muscles in the stomatognathic system [6], and symptoms related to OMD include masticatory disturbances, limited mouth opening, muscle pain, dysphagia, dysarthria, esthetic problems, and temporomandibular joint dislocation [6,10]. Bakke [Contribution 6] provided a review that introduced BoNT as a medical treatment for conditions of the orofacial region and focused on OMD and sialorrhea after supplementary training and according to the national guidelines, as these are relevant to dentists and also emphasized the need for interdisciplinary collaboration between dentists, neurologists and/or otologists for precise diagnostics and treatment. To achieve the best results and minimize or prevent side effects, standard doses should be used. Moreover, guidance on BoNT injections with electromyography or ultrasonography should be considered and regular and standardized treatments and controls should be investigated in future [Contribution 6]. The symptoms of OMD, such as jaw closing, jaw opening, and tongue dystonia, vary considerably according to the subtypes. In a follow-up questionnaire 8–10 years after the start of repeated BoNT treatment, which was answered by 14 persons with OMD, nine were still being treated with BoNT injections 3–4 times per year as monotherapy or combined with oral medication [7]. The most often reported dystonic symptoms were jaw closing and opening, as well as munching and chewing movements. In particular, eating and mental stress were reported to increase the dystonic activity, and sleep, relaxation, and quietness to decrease it. Most of the respondents felt that the BoNT treatment relieved their symptoms and the change of score a VAS scale for OMD symptoms was significant, with a reduction of 16%, either as an effect of the repeated BoNT injections or due to the time course [7]. Yoshida [Contribution 7] evaluated 408 patients [jaw closing dystonia, $n = 223$; tongue (lingual) dystonia, $n = 86$; jaw opening dystonia, $n = 50$; jaw deviation dystonia, $n = 23$; jaw protrusion dystonia, $n = 13$; and lip (labial) dystonia, $n = 13$] at baseline and after the end of BoNT therapy or in a stable status. All examiner-rated subscales (severity, disability, and pain) and patient-rated questionnaire scores (general, eating, speech, cosmetic, social/family life, sleep, annoyance, mood, and psychosocial function) were significantly lower at the endpoint than at baseline ($p < 0.001$). BoNT injection positively impacted the health-related quality of life, and the rating scale could evaluate both motor phenomena and non-motor symptoms when properly diagnosed and administered precisely. The rating scale can be used to comprehensively evaluate both therapeutic effects and health-related quality of life. Bilateral brain stimulation has been applied for the treatment of OMD, yet, for some patients, the symptoms do not improve sufficiently and additional BoNT injections may be required.

In clinical dentistry or oral surgery, we often encounter patients with orolingual dyskinesia or tardive syndrome. Skarmeta et al. [Contribution 8] reported a rare case with Trazodone, a (tetracyclic antidepressant)-induced OMD. Early identification and assessment of tardive symptoms are imperative for successful treatment, and Trazodone should be prescribed with caution in patients taking other medications with the potential to cause tardive syndromes. Preventing and identifying the onset of tardive syndromes is of paramount importance, and the authors suggested that clinicians should balance the risk/benefit ratio before prescribing drugs that can potentially produce tardive symptoms.

The cosmetic use of BoNT in clinical practice is significant. It is an important and interesting field for many clinicians and patients and there has been a global rise in the demand for non-invasive procedures to help patients rejuvenate their appearance. BoNT is now the most performed esthetic procedure in the world and various types of BoNT with different properties have become available. Hong provided an excellent practical illustrative guide and reference for BoNT applications in the orofacial area including safe injection areas and effective doses [Contribution 9]. To ensure safety and effectiveness, appropriate guidelines on the use of BoNT injections for the treatment of dynamic rhytides and hypertrophic structure is warranted.

This Special Issue is representative of dental professionals who use BoNT injections worldwide, with contributors who are specialists in the relevant fields, producing papers that examined the treatment's effectiveness and safety. However, the approved indications for BoNT injections may vary between countries and, to be officially approved for a certain indication, evidence from well-designed, randomized, controlled trials with larger sample sizes and longer follow-up periods are essential. If the number of experts in each country is limited, international collaborative research may be necessary. To facilitate the use of BoNT widely and routinely by general practitioners guidelines for safe and effective treatment must be established.

BoNT is very expensive, meaning that there is a possibility that some clinicians will overlook conventional treatment methods and use BoNT instead for profit. Consequently, the medical costs may skyrocket. Therefore, supplementary training or some kind of qualification should be the basic requirement for using BoNT therapeutically. In addition, differential diagnosis is important for neurological diseases, such as OMD, and collaboration between neurological and dental experts is advisable [Contributions 5–7]. Since dental professionals are specialists of the stomatognathic system, they, rather than medical professionals, may have the skills to provide more accurate injections to target the muscles of interest in the oral region. Ultimately, effective and safe BoNT therapy requires a multidisciplinary team approach.

Author Contributions: K.Y. and M.B. wrote and revised the manuscript. All authors have read and agreed to the published version of the manuscript.

Conflicts of Interest: The authors declare no conflicts of interest.

List of Contributions:

1. De la Torre Canales, G.; Poluha, R.L.; Pinzón, N.A.; Da Silva, B.R.; Almeida, A.M.; Ernberg, M.; Manso, A.C.; Bonjardim, L.R.; Rizzatti-Barbosa, C.M. Efficacy of botulinum toxin type-A I in the improvement of mandibular motion and muscle sensibility in myofascial pain TMD subjects: A randomized controlled trial. *Toxins* **2022**, *14*, 441. https://doi.org/10.3390/toxins14070441.
2. De la Torre Canales, G.; Câmara-Souza, M.B.; Poluha, R.L.; de Figueredo, O.M.C.; Nobre, B.B.d.S.; Ernberg, M.; Conti, P.C.R.; Rizzatti-Barbosa, C.M. Long-term effects of a single application of botulinum toxin type A in temporomandibular myofascial pain patients: A controlled clinical trial. *Toxins* **2022**, *14*, 741. https://doi.org/10.3390/toxins14110741.
3. Sitnikova, V.; Kämppi, A.; Teronen, O.; Kemppainen, P. Effect of botulinum toxin injection on EMG activity and bite force in masticatory muscle disorder: A randomized clinical trial. *Toxins* **2022**, *14*, 545. https://doi.org/10.3390/toxins14080545.
4. Val, M.; Delcanho, R.; Ferrari, M.; Guarda Nardini, L.; Manfredini, D. Is botulinum toxin effective in treating orofacial neuropathic pain disorders? A systematic review. *Toxins* **2023**, *15*, 541. https://doi.org/10.3390/toxins15090541.
5. Kępczyńska, K.; Domitrz, I. Botulinum toxin—A current place in the treatment of chronic migraine and other primary headaches. *Toxins* **2022**, *14*, 619. https://doi.org/10.3390/toxins14090619.
6. Bakke, M. Botulinum toxin, a drug with potential interest for dentists—An introduction. *Toxins* **2022**, *14*, 667. https://doi.org/10.3390/toxins14100667.
7. Yoshida, K. Effects of botulinum toxin therapy on health-related quality of life evaluated by the oromandibular dystonia rating scale. *Toxins* **2022**, *14*, 656. https://doi.org/10.3390/toxins14100656.
8. Skarmeta, N.P.; Katzmann, G.C.; Valdés, C.; Gaedechens, D.; Montini, F.C. Tardive oromandibular dystonia induced by Trazodone: A clinical case and management from the perspective of the dental specialist. *Toxins* **2022**, *14*, 680. https://doi.org/10.3390/toxins14100680.
9. Hong, S.O. Cosmetic treatment using botulinum toxin in the oral and maxillofacial area: A narrative review of esthetic techniques. *Toxins* **2023**, *15*, 82. https://doi.org/10.3390/toxins15020082.

References

1. Kerner, J. *Vergiftung durch verdorbene Wurste. Tübinger Blätter für Naturwissenschaften und Arzneykunde*; C.F. Osiander: Tübingen, Germany, 1817; Volume 3, pp. 1–25.
2. Van Ermengem, E. Über eine neuen anaeroben Bacillus und seine Beziehungen zum Botulismus. *Z. Hyg. Infektionskrankh.* **1897**, *26*, 1–56.
3. Scott, A.B. Botulinum toxin injection into extraocular muscles as an alternative to strabismus surgery. *Opthalmology* **1980**, *87*, 1044–1049. [CrossRef] [PubMed]
4. Hallett, M.; Albanese, A.; Dressler, D.; Segal, K.R.; Simpson, D.M.; Truong, D.; Jankovic, J. Evidence-based review and assessment of botulinum neurotoxin for the treatment of movement disorders. *Toxicon* **2013**, *67*, 94–114. [CrossRef] [PubMed]
5. Anandan, C.; Jankovic, J. Botulinum toxin in movement disorders: An update. *Toxins* **2021**, *13*, 42. [CrossRef] [PubMed]
6. Yoshida, K. Botulinum toxin therapy for oromandibular dystonia and other movement disorders in the stomatognathic system. *Toxins* **2022**, *14*, 282. [CrossRef] [PubMed]
7. Bakke, M.; Baram, S.; Dalager, T.; Biernat, H.B.; Møller, E. Oromandibular dystonia, mental distress and oro-facial dysfunction—A follow-up 8–10 years after start of treatment with botulinum toxin. *J. Oral Rehabil.* **2019**, *46*, 441–449. [CrossRef] [PubMed]
8. Ernberg, M.; Hedenberg-Magnusson, B.; List, T.; Svensson, P. Efficacy of botulinum toxin type A for treatment of persistent myofascial TMD pain: A randomized, controlled, double-blind multicenter study. *Pain* **2011**, *152*, 1988–1996. [CrossRef] [PubMed]

9. Schiffman, E.; Ohrbach, R.; Truelove, E.; Look, J.; Anderson, G.; Goulet, J.P. Diagnostic Criteria for TMD (DC/TMD) for Clinical and Research Applications: Recommendations of the International RDC/TMD Consortium Network and Orofacial Pain Special Interest Group. *J. Orofac. Pain.* **2014**, *28*, 6–27. [CrossRef]
10. Scorr, L.M.; Factor, S.A.; Parra, S.P.; Kaye, R.; Paniello, R.C.; Norris, S.A.; Perlmutter, J.S.; Bäumer, T.; Usnich, T.; Berman, B.D.; et al. Oromandibular dystonia: A clinical examination of 2020 cases. *Front. Neurol.* **2021**, *12*, 700714. [CrossRef] [PubMed]

toxins

MDPI

Article

Long-Term Effects of a Single Application of Botulinum Toxin Type A in Temporomandibular Myofascial Pain Patients: A Controlled Clinical Trial

Giancarlo De la Torre Canales [1,2,3,*], Mariana Barbosa Câmara-Souza [2,3], Rodrigo Lorenzi Poluha [4], Olívia Maria Costa de Figueredo [3], Bryanne Brissian de Souza Nobre [2], Malin Ernberg [5], Paulo César Rodrigues Conti [6] and Célia Marisa Rizzatti-Barbosa [2,3]

1 Clinical Research Unit (CRU), Centro de Investigação Interdisciplinar Egas Moniz (CiiEM), Egas Moniz, Cooperativa de Ensino Superior, CRL, 2829-511 Caparica, Portugal
2 Ingá University Center, Uningá, Paraná 87015-510, Brazil
3 Department of Prosthodontics and Periodontology, Piracicaba Dental School, University of Campinas, Piracicaba, São Paulo 13414-903, Brazil
4 Department of Dentistry, State University of Maringa, Paraná 87020-900, Brazil
5 Department of Dental Medicine, Karolinska Institutet, and the Scandinavian Center for Orofacial Neurosciences (SCON), 141 52 Huddinge, Sweden
6 Bauru Orofacial Pain Group, Department of Prosthodontics, Bauru School of Dentistry, University of São Paulo, São Paulo 17012-900, Brazil
* Correspondence: giank_28@hotmail.com; Tel.: +5519-9714-15148

Abstract: This study assessed the long-term effects of botulinum toxin type A (BoNT-A) in subjective pain, pain sensibility, and muscle thickness in persistent myofascial temporomandibular-disorder pain (MFP-TMD) patients. Fourteen female subjects with persistent MFP received BoNT-A treatment with different doses (10U-25U for temporalis muscle and 30U-75U for masseter muscle). The treatment was injected bilaterally in the masseter and anterior temporalis muscles in a single session. Clinical measurements included: self-perceived pain (VAS), pain sensibility (PPT), and muscles thickness (ultrasonography). Follow-up occurred 1, 3, 6, and 72 months after treatment for VAS and PPT and 1, 3, and 72 months for ultrasonography. For statistical analysis, the Friedman test with the Bonferroni test for multiple comparisons as a post hoc test was used for non-parametric repeated measures comparisons among the evaluation times. A 5% probability level was considered significant in all tests. VAS values presented a significant decrease throughout the study ($p < 0.05$). Regarding PPT values, a significant increase was found when comparing baseline data with post-treatment follow-ups ($p < 0.05$), and even though a significant decrease was found in muscle thickness when baseline values were compared with the 1- and 3-months assessments, no differences were found when compared with the 72 months follow-up ($p > 0.05$). A single injection of BoNT-A presents long-term effects in reducing pain in persistent MFP-TMD patients, and a reversibility of adverse effects on masticatory-muscle thickness.

Keywords: botulinum toxin type A; myofascial pain; temporomandibular disorders; muscle thickness

Key Contribution: A single injection of BoNT-A could be considered a safe and effective treatment for persistent MFP patients since it has long-term beneficial therapeutic effects and presents a reversibility of adverse effects in masticatory muscles.

Citation: De la Torre Canales, G.; Câmara-Souza, M.B.; Poluha, R.L.; de Figueredo, O.M.C.; Nobre, B.B.d.S.; Ernberg, M.; Conti, P.C.R.; Rizzatti-Barbosa, C.M. Long-Term Effects of a Single Application of Botulinum Toxin Type A in Temporomandibular Myofascial Pain Patients: A Controlled Clinical Trial. *Toxins* **2022**, *14*, 741. https://doi.org/10.3390/toxins14110741

Received: 7 October 2022
Accepted: 28 October 2022
Published: 29 October 2022

1. Introduction

Myofascial pain (MFP) has been related to affect up to 95% of patients with chronic pain [1] and is reported by 45% of those with temporomandibular disorders (TMD) [2]. This condition is characterized by local and referred pain, muscle stiffness, and sensory changes, with a multifactorial etiology.

Considering its high prevalence and chronicity, multidisciplinary approaches have been suggested for treatment. Although non-invasive conservative treatments should be considered as the first-choice intervention [3], dealing with chronic pain conditions demands investigating new modalities to reduce symptomatology and provide quality of life. Therefore, botulinum toxin type A (BoNT-A) was introduced to be used in a variety of chronic pain conditions due to its antinociceptive effect, being reported to suppress neurotransmitters secretion, thereby decreasing peripheral and central sensitization [4,5].

Several studies have reported the positive effects of BoNT-A in pain syndromes [6], such as neuropathic pain [7], chronic migraine [8,9], trigeminal neuralgia [10], chronic back pain [11], chronic pelvic pain [12], and chronic myofascial pain in TMD patients [13]. Considering its use for TMD management, our/a previous study [13] has shown reduction in patient-reported pain and pain sensitivity, demonstrating BoNT-A's positive effect for this condition. However, adverse effects were also reported, for example, worsened masticatory performance, decreased muscle thickness, and reduction in mandibular bone volume [13]. Such outcomes are mainly related to muscle paralysis, which led to changes in muscle and bone morphologies, that could, ultimately, impair daily activities.

However, studies evaluating improvements and adverse effects after BoNT-A's applications in muscle pain conditions are limited to short-term follow-ups, which jeopardize findings regarding effectiveness [13]. In addition, no study has assessed if the reported adverse effects produced by BoNT-A are permanent or reversible. Therefore, the present study aimed to investigate the long-term effects of one single injection of BoNT-A on masticatory muscles, after 6 years, in patients with persistent MFP-TMD. The null hypothesis is that after all these years, no beneficial or negative effects should be found, with patients presenting pain scores and muscle thickness resembling the initial appointment.

2. Results

From the initial 60 patients treated with BoNT-A, 14 individuals (23%) returned for the 6-year assessment (Figure 1). Even though some investigators assessing the outcomes after 6 years of follow-up were different from the original study, interclass correlation (ICC) showed an excellent inter-rater reliability for all variables (0.912 for subjective pain intensity; 0.910 for pressure-pain threshold; and 0.915 for muscle thickness) [13].

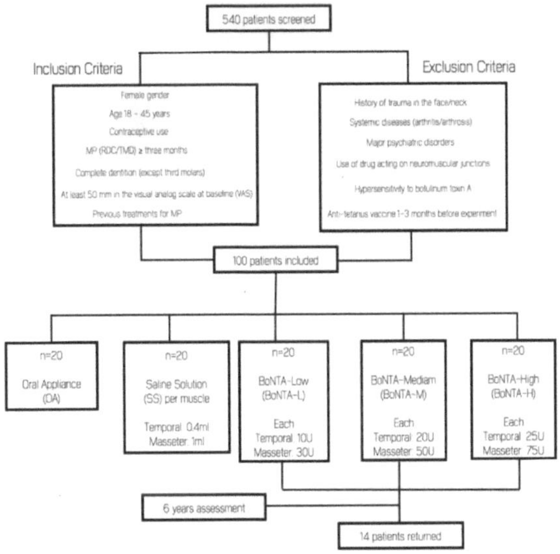

Figure 1. Flow diagram of patient's recruitment.

2.1. *Self-Perceived Pain: Visual Analog Scale (VAS)*

Compared to the baseline data, a significant decrease of subjective pain was already found one month after treatment ($p < 0.001$). This pain reduction was maintained in subsequent examinations, with no significant differences until the 6-year evaluation ($p > 0.05$) (Table 1).

Table 1. Median, minimum, and maximum values for subjective pain intensity (mm) in 14 patients with temporomandibular-disorder myofascial pain before and at different time-points after a single-injection of botulinum toxin.

	Time				
	Baseline	**1 Month**	**3 Months**	**6 Months**	**6 Years**
Median	7.85	1.15 *	0.00 *	0.00 *	0.30*
Minimum	5.90	0.00	0.00	0.00	0.00
Maximum	10.00	7.10	5.60	6.60	8.10

* Significant difference compared to baseline ($p < 0.05$; Friedman test with Bonferroni test for multiple comparisons as posthoc test).

2.2. *Pain Sensitivity: Pressure-Pain Threshold (PPT)*

In the PPT evaluation for both muscles, there was no difference between the baseline data and the one-month evaluation ($p > 0.05$). However, after three months there was a significant increase in PPT's values compared with the baseline and the one-month assessment period ($p < 0.001$) (Table 2). This significant difference remained until the last evaluation period, with no significant difference between the last three periods of assessment.

Table 2. Median, minimum, and maximum values for pressure-pain threshold (Kg/f) in 14 patients with temporomandibular-disorder myofascial pain before and at different time-points after a single-injection of botulinum toxin.

		Time				
		Baseline	**1 Month**	**3 Months**	**6 Months**	**6 Years**
Anterior Temporalis	Median	0.51	0.89	1.02 *	1.22 *	1.18 *
	Minimum	0.30	0.26	0.32	0.45	0.56
	Maximum	0.75	1.44	1.62	1.62	2.05
Masseter	Median	0.45	0.85	0.95 *	1.07 *	1.03 *
	Minimum	0.26	0.29	0.32	0.44	0.53
	Maximum	0.79	1.42	1.54	1.28	2.03

* Significant difference compared to baseline ($p < 0.05$; Friedman test with Bonferroni test for multiple comparisons as posthoc test).

2.3. *Ultrasound Imaging*

Masseters and anterior temporalis muscles thickness during maximum volunteer contraction decreased after BoNT-A application, even after the first month ($p < 0.001$). Although this reduction remained after 3 months, at the 6-year period it was not possible to observe any statistically significant difference from the baseline (Table 3).

Table 3. Median, minimum, and maximum values for muscle thickness (mm) in 14 patients with temporomandibular-disorder myofascial pain before and at different time-points after a single-session treatment with botulinum toxin.

		Time			
		Baseline	**1 Month**	**3 Months**	**6 Years**
Anterior Temporalis	Median	2.02	1.30 *	1.38 *	2.15
	Minimum	0.80	0.80	0.90	1.30
	Maximum	1.70	3.20	2.40	3.40
Masseter	Median	12.52	10.42 *	11.37 *	13.20
	Minimum	9.95	7.60	8.95	12.00
	Maximum	12.35	12.70	12.45	15.60

* Significant difference compared to baseline ($p < 0.05$; Friedman test with Bonferroni test for multiple comparisons as posthoc test).

3. Discussion

To the best of the authors' knowledge, this is the first clinical trial to demonstrate the improvement of pain features and the reversibility of masticatory muscles adverse effects, after a 6-year follow-up of a single injection of BoNT-A regardless of dosage, in persistent MFP TMD patients. The results showed that BoNT-A produced a significant reduction in subjective pain after the first month of evaluation, which remained until the 6-year evaluation. Likewise, BoNT-A increased PPT values of masticatory muscles since the third month of assessment, which lasted up to the 6-year follow-up. Conversely, even though BoNT-A decreased muscle thickness (an adverse effect) in the first two periods of evaluation, after 6 years there was masticatory-muscle thickness recovery.

The positive effects of BoNT-A in a variety of chronic pain conditions [5] have been reported by some well-designed clinical trials [7,8,10]. In addition, in vivo and in vitro studies have reported that the antinociceptive effect of BoNT-A is mainly related to a peripheral and central decrease of neurotransmitters such as glutamate, substance P, and calcitonin-gene-related peptide (CGRP) [14–16], and by its axonal transport to sensory regions of the trigeminal ganglion [17,18], the modulation of the spinal opioidergic or GABA-ergic system [19,20], and the prevention of microglia activation [21,22]. However, despite the fact that several clinical trials [23–28] have assessed BoNT-A efficacy for myofascial pain relief, its efficacy has not yet been established. Methodological shortcomings may explain the conflicting results.

Our findings showed that a single injection of BoNT-A, regardless of the dose, already produced a significant improvement in terms of subjective pain after one month of evaluation and was sustained until the 6-year evaluation. Our findings are in line with reports demonstrating a decrease in subjective pain after BoNT-A injection in samples with the same characteristics as ours after 4 [26] and 6 [28] months of follow-up. Additionally, our study found that PPT values significantly increased after 3 months of assessment and that this effect was maintained until the 6-year follow-up. Likewise, previous studies [23,26,29] have shown that BoNT-A was able to diminish muscle tenderness to palpation when compared to the placebo over 3 to 6 months. On the other hand, a doble-blind crossover study [24] including the same population characteristics as ours showed that while BoNT-A achieved a clinically significant reduction in subjective pain (i.e., 30% less pain), no differences were found when compared with the placebo group after three months of evaluation of subjective pain intensity and PPT assessment. Perhaps the differences in the methodology, such as treating just one muscle group (masseter), may have influenced the results.

Moreover, one question remains unclear about the BoNT-A analgesic mechanism of action: is it predominantly peripheric or central? There is plenty of literature about the analgesic peripheral effects of BoNT-A [5]; however, the evidence and research about BoNT-A analgesic effects are increasing, leading to the proposal of new pathways that BoNT-A can use in order to reach the central nervous system. In animals, it was demonstrated that BoNT-

A inhibits central nociceptor transduction and central neurotransmitter release [21,30]. In fact, a clinical trial involving neuropathic pain patients (chronic pain condition) showed pain improvement after BoNT-A injections, although the quantity of the neurotransmitter in the biopsies of painful regions remained high. Based on these results, the authors proposed that the analgesic effect of BoNT-A is mainly related to the central mechanisms of pain transmission, at least in chronic pain conditions. Since MFP is also considered a chronic condition, this hypothesis could also be applied to our positive results. Notwithstanding, it is also known that persistent MFP-TMD patients present a deficit in pain modulation [31]. Considering that BoNT-A modulates the opioidergic and GABA-ergic systems [19,20], its effects on pain modulation could also explain the long-term effects presented in our study, corroborating the later hypothesis.

BoNT-A treatment is considered generally safe because the doses used for pain conditions are far from the lethal doses. In addition, a systematic review [27] reported that this treatment is generally tolerated since self-reported minor adverse effects (e.g., short-term facial weakness, pain at the injection site, transient edema, and minimum discomfort during chewing) that resolved spontaneously were the most prevalent. However, the authors [27] also concluded that none of the included studies aimed to assess objectively adverse effects on muscle and bone tissue. Notwithstanding, in the last few years some clinical and experimental [27,32,33] studies have reported "severe" adverse effects of BoNT-A, which include masticatory muscle atrophy and the loss of mandibular bone volume. Our study confirmed literature findings since a significant reduction in masticatory muscle thickness was found after 1 and 3 months of injection, independent of dosage.

The reduction in muscle thickness is part of a series of events produced when BoNT-A is injected. First, a muscle paralysis is caused by a neural denervation that lasts for at least three months [34], during which new nerve fibers are produced to innervate the muscular portion that was paralyzed; however, it was demonstrated that these new motor fibers do not have enough potency to innervate the muscle effectively. Then, the lack of sufficient innervation causes structural changes in masticatory muscles, including the diminution of the quantity of muscle fibers [32], changes in the quality of remnant muscle fibers [32], the reduction in muscle-fiber size [33], the replacement of contractile tissue with fat [35], and an increase in the mRNA expression of muscle-atrophy markers [33]. Finally, as a result of all of the structural changes after BoNT-A injection, a decrease in muscle thickness is produced. Nevertheless, our study found that the decrease in muscle thickness seems to be reversable since significant muscle thickness recovery was found in masseter and anterior temporalis muscles after the 6-year follow-up, showing no differences with baseline data. This finding allows us to suggest that the recovery of masticatory-muscle thickness is not related to the units of BoNT-A injected, but it could be related to the number of times that BoNT-A is injected, as concluded by Rauso et al. (2022) [36]. A prospective interventional trial of patients receiving a protocol of three repeated cycles of 30U (considered in our study as low dosage) of BoNT-A for masseter hypertrophy for 6 months demonstrated a dramatic reduction in muscle thickness (42.52%) after a follow-up of 35 weeks, which was sustained after a 4-year follow-up [37]. This result supports the cumulative adverse effect of repeated cycles of low doses of BoNT-A on muscle thickness, which could be considered irreversible.

Although our results demonstrated positive effects of a single injection of BoNT-A regardless of the dose, caution is suggested when judging the present findings since some limitations should be mentioned. The present study was performed on a convenience population, without sex comparison. Additionally, although the rate of patients who returned to the 6-year follow-up could be considered acceptable (23%), a larger sample size is required for future studies. Additionally, it cannot be excluded that factors such as the placebo effect, the natural evolution of the disease (myofascial TMD pain), and the regression toward the mean may also partially explain treatment outcomes. However, it is important to mention that the study population was composed of persistent MFP TMD patients that had suffered for at least 6 months [13], and that BoNT-A was the only treatment that produced a significant improvement in their perceived pain. Moreover, it should be considered that patients could have received other treatments during the last 6 years; in fact, most of them reported that only self-care strategies to control pain (thermotheraphy and massage in the painful area) were used. Additionally, the risk of sample bias cannot be excluded, i.e., that the study population was mainly composed of patients that experienced significant positive effects after the BoNT-A injections performed in our previous study, a fact that certainly could have influenced the favorable effects reported in the present study. We recommend assessing the reversibility of adverse effects on bone tissues after a single injection of BoNT-A since it is related to changes in muscle tissues. Finally, future studies should assess the clinically meaningful adverse effects on muscle and bone tissue arising from multiple applications of BoNT-A, and especially their reversibility.

4. Conclusions

Based on the results and limitations of this study, and considering the possible placebo effects on pain variable, it can be concluded that:

A single injection of BoNT-A, regardless of dosage, could present long-term effects in reducing pain in persistent MFP TMD patients, that did not achieve significant pain relief using conservative therapies.

There is a reversibility of adverse effects on masticatory-muscle thickness after a single injection of BoNT-A, which may be related to the number of times that the toxin is injected and not to the doses.

5. Methods

5.1. Subjects

The present clinical trial reports the 6-year follow-up results of a previous study [13] performed with 100 persistent MFP-TMD female subjects. The former study included BoNT-A injection, oral appliance (positive control), and saline solution (placebo) groups, and assessed outcomes before treatment and after 1, 3, and 6 months. Participants were recruited from women seeking TMD treatment at the TMD Clinic of Piracicaba Dental School, University of Campinas, São Paulo, Brazil. Patients were diagnosed according to the Portuguese version of the Research Diagnostic Criteria for Temporomandibular Disorders [38] by two calibrated researchers not involved in any other processes of the study (kappa coefficient = 0.80). The study was approved by the Research Ethics Committee of Piracicaba Dental School (CAAE # 22953113.8.0000.5418-Date: 4 February 2014) and the Brazilian Registry of Clinical Trials (ReBEC RBR-2d4vvv). All subjects were informed about the research purposes and provided written informed consent to participate in this clinical trial. Inclusion and exclusion criteria have been previously detailed [13].

Therefore, subjects included in the present study were a convenience sample of the study of De la Torre Canales et al. (2020) [13], which assessed the efficacy and adverse effects of different doses of BoNT-A up to six months of follow-up. Since the primary objective of this study was to assess the reversibility of adverse effects, the positive (splint) and negative (saline solution) control groups were not included, due to the absence of statistically significance differences in the previous one [13]. Therefore, only participants assigned to the BoNT-A groups (n = 60) were contacted. The patients were recruited via telephone for the 6-year assessment.

5.2. Treatments

BoNT-A (100 U; Botox, Allergan, Irvine, California, CA, USA) was reconstituted using non-preserved sterile saline solution 0.9%. Bilateral intramuscular injections were performed using a 1 mL syringe with a 30-gauge and 13 mm needle. For each masseter muscle, doses from 30U to 75U were distributed in five sites 5 mm apart from each other and were injected in the inferior part of the muscle (on mandibular angle) after functional test (teeth clenching). For each anterior temporalis muscle, doses from 10U to 25U were distributed in five sites 5 mm apart from each other, which were determined according to the functional test considering the most prominent part, which had to be 1 cm external to the eyebrow. Injections were performed by a calibrated researcher during a single appointment.

6. Primary Outcomes

6.1. Self-Perceived Pain: Visual Analog Scale

A visual analogue scale (VAS) [39] is a 100 mm horizontal line, anchored by the words "no pain" at the left end and "worst pain imaginable" at the right end. Participants were instructed to mark a line at any point representing the level of their current, worst, and average pain of the last month. Mean values were used for statistical analyses.

6.2. Pain sensitivity: Pressure-Pain Threshold

Pressure-pain thresholds (PPT) [40] was measured using a digital algometer (model DDK- 20, Kratos®, Cotia, São Paulo, Brazil). The algometer has a 1-cm^2 flat circular-shaped tip at one end, which was used to apply pressure to the most prominent part (determined with functional test) of the relaxed masseter and anterior temporalis muscles. The device was positioned perpendicularly to the muscles and applied with increasing and constant pressure of approximately 0.5 kgf/cm^2 by a new single calibrated operator (Kappa = 0.89), which was blind for the injected groups. Patients were asked to press a button at the very beginning of pain sensation. The procedure was fully explained to each patient before the examination, and it was emphasized that the purpose of the study was to measure the PPT and not pain tolerance. PPT measurement sites were aligned with BoNT-A injections sites. The PPT was determined as the arithmetic mean of three measurements.

7. Secondary Outcome

7.1. Ultrasound Imaging

The thickness of both masseters and anterior temporalis muscles during maximum voluntary contraction (MVC) was calculated using real-time ultrasound imaging (UI; SSA-780 A-APLIO Mx, 38 mm/7-18 MHz; Toshiba Medical SystemCo., Tokyo, Japan). A different calibrated operator performed the 6-year measurement. The patients were placed in a supine position at a height that ergonomically favored the examination. Muscle thickness was measured directly on the instrument's screen, with an accuracy of 0.01 mm according to the most voluminous part of the muscle in the screen image. UI values were determined as the arithmetic mean of three measurements [41].

7.2. Data Evaluation and Statistical Analyses

Subjective pain intensity (VAS) and PPT were assessed at five-time points: before treatment (baseline) and at one, three, and six months, as well as six years after treatment. Data from muscle thickness, measured with ultrasound imaging, were assessed at four-time points: before treatment (baseline), one and three months after treatment, and six years after treatment. The inter-rater reliability was assessed by the Intraclass correlation coefficient (ICC). The Kolmogorov–Smirnov test demonstrated no normal distribution. Then, the Friedman test with the Bonferroni test for multiple comparisons as a posthoc test was used for non-parametric repeated measures comparisons among the evaluation times. All data were analyzed using SPSS Statistics 25.0 software (IBM®, New York, NY, USA). A 5% probability level was considered significant in all tests.

Author Contributions: Conceptualization, G.D.l.T.C., M.B.C.-S., R.L.P., O.M.C.d.F. and C.M.R.-B.; data curation, G.D.l.T.C., M.B.C.-S., R.L.P., O.M.C.d.F. and B.B.d.S.N.; formal analysis, R.L.P., C.M.R.-B., P.C.R.C. and M.E.; funding acquisition, G.D.l.T.C. and C.M.R.-B.; investigation, G.D.l.T.C., M.B.C.-S. and O.M.C.d.F.; methodology, G.D.l.T.C., M.B.C.-S., R.L.P., O.M.C.d.F., B.B.d.S.N., M.E., P.C.R.C. and C.M.R.-B.; project administration, G.D.l.T.C., M.E., P.C.R.C. and C.M.R.-B.; writing—original draft, G.D.l.T.C., M.B.C.-S., R.L.P. and B.B.d.S.N.; and writing—review and editing, G.D.l.T.C., M.B.C.-S., R.L.P., O.M.C.d.F., B.B.d.S.N., M.E., P.C.R.C. and C.M.R.-B. All authors have read and agreed to the published version of the manuscript.

Funding: This study was financed by the Sao Paulo Research Foundation (FAPESP)—Brazil (grant number 2014/15863-7).

Institutional Review Board Statement: The study was conducted according to the guidelines of the Declaration of Helsinki and approved by the Ethics Committee of Piracicaba Dental School—University of Campinas (CAAE # 22953113.8.0000.5418—Date: 4 February 2014).

Informed Consent Statement: Informed consent was obtained from all subjects involved in the study.

Data Availability Statement: The data presented in this study are available in this article.

Acknowledgments: We acknowledge the Coordenação de Aperfeiçoamento de Pessoal de Nível Superior—Brasil (CAPES) Finance Code 001 for the Ph.D. scholarship of R. Lorenzi Poluha, the Sao Paulo Research Foundation (FAPESP)—Brazil for the Post-Doctoral scholarship of G. De la Torre Canales (process 2017/21674-0), and the Ph.D. scholarship of M. B. Câmara-Souza (process 2017/23429-3).

Conflicts of Interest: The funding sources were not involved in the study design; the collection, analysis, or interpretation of data; the decision to publish; or the preparation of the manuscript. The authors declare no conflict of interest.

References

1. Nasirzadeh, Y.; Ahmed, S.; Monteiro, S.; Grosman-Rimon, L.; Srbely, J.; Kumbhare, D. A survey of healthcare practitioners on myofascial pain criteria. *Pain Pract.* **2018**, *18*, 631–640. [CrossRef]
2. Manfredini, D.; Ahlberg, J.; Winocur, E.; Guarda-Nardini, L.; Lobbezoo, F. Correlation of RDC/TMD axis I diagnoses and axis II pain-related disability. A multicenter study. *Clin. Oral Investig.* **2011**, *15*, 749–756. [CrossRef]
3. Reid, K.; Greene, C. Diagnosis and treatment of temporomandibular disorders: An ethical analysis of current practices. *J. Oral Rehabil.* **2013**, *40*, 546–561. [CrossRef] [PubMed]
4. Arezzo, J.C. Possible mechanisms for the effects of botulinum toxin on pain. *Clin. J. Pain* **2002**, *18*, S125–S132. [CrossRef]
5. Matak, I.; Bölcskei, K.; Bach-Rojecky, L.; Helyes, Z. Mechanisms of botulinum toxin type A action on pain. *Toxins* **2019**, *11*, 459. [CrossRef] [PubMed]
6. Safarpour, Y.; Jabbari, B. Botulinum toxin treatment of pain syndromes–an evidence based review. *Toxicon* **2018**, *147*, 120–128. [CrossRef]
7. Attal, N.; de Andrade, D.C.; Adam, F.; Ranoux, D.; Teixeira, M.J.; Galhardoni, R.; Raicher, I.; Üçeyler, N.; Sommer, C.; Bouhassira, D. Safety and efficacy of repeated injections of botulinum toxin A in peripheral neuropathic pain (BOTNEP): A randomised, double-blind, placebo-controlled trial. *Lancet Neurol.* **2016**, *15*, 555–565. [CrossRef]
8. Diener, H.; Dodick, D.; Aurora, S.; Turkel, C.; DeGryse, R.; Lipton, R.; Silberstein, S.; Brin, M. OnabotulinumtoxinA for treatment of chronic migraine: Results from the double-blind, randomized, placebo-controlled phase of the PREEMPT 2 trial. *Cephalalgia* **2010**, *30*, 804–814. [CrossRef]
9. Luvisetto, S.; Gazerani, P.; Cianchetti, C.; Pavone, F. Botulinum toxin type a as a therapeutic agent against headache and related disorders. *Toxins* **2015**, *7*, 3818–3844. [CrossRef]
10. Zhang, H.; Lian, Y.; Ma, Y.; Chen, Y.; He, C.; Xie, N.; Wu, C. Two doses of botulinum toxin type A for the treatment of trigeminal neuralgia: Observation of therapeutic effect from a randomized, double-blind, placebo-controlled trial. *J. Headache Pain* **2014**, *15*, 65. [CrossRef]
11. Foster, L.; Clapp, L.; Erickson, M.; Jabbari, B. Botulinum toxin A and chronic low back pain: A randomized, double-blind study. *Neurology* **2001**, *56*, 1290–1293. [CrossRef] [PubMed]
12. Chen, C.-L.; Meng, E. Can botulinum toxin A play a role in treatment of chronic pelvic pain syndrome in female patients?—Clinical and animal evidence. *Toxins* **2020**, *12*, 110. [CrossRef] [PubMed]
13. De la Torre Canales, G.; Alvarez-Pinzon, N.; Muñoz-Lora, V.R.M.; Vieira Peroni, L.; Farias Gomes, A.; Sánchez-Ayala, A.; Haiter-Neto, F.; Manfredini, D.; Rizzatti-Barbosa, C.M. Efficacy and safety of botulinum toxin type a on persistent myofascial pain: A randomized clinical trial. *Toxins* **2020**, *12*, 395. [CrossRef]
14. Purkiss, J.; Welch, M.; Doward, S.; Foster, K. Capsaicin-stimulated release of substance P from cultured dorsal root ganglion neurons: Involvement of two distinct mechanisms. *Biochem. Pharmacol.* **2000**, *59*, 1403–1406. [CrossRef]
15. Cui, M.; Khanijou, S.; Rubino, J.; Aoki, K.R. Subcutaneous administration of botulinum toxin A reduces formalin-induced pain. *Pain* **2004**, *107*, 125–133. [CrossRef] [PubMed]
16. Lora, V.R.M.M.; Clemente-Napimoga, J.T.; Abdalla, H.B.; Macedo, C.G.; de la Torre Canales, G.; Barbosa, C.M.R. Botulinum toxin type A reduces inflammatory hypernociception induced by arthritis in the temporomadibular joint of rats. *Toxicon* **2017**, *129*, 52–57. [CrossRef]
17. Bach-Rojecky, L.; Lacković, Z. Central origin of the antinociceptive action of botulinum toxin type A. *Pharmacol. Biochem. Behav.* **2009**, *94*, 234–238. [CrossRef]

18. Matak, I.; Bach-Rojecky, L.; Filipović, B.; Lacković, Z. Behavioral and immunohistochemical evidence for central antinociceptive activity of botulinum toxin A. *Neuroscience* **2011**, *186*, 201–207. [CrossRef]
19. Drinovac, V.; Bach-Rojecky, L.; Matak, I.; Lacković, Z. Involvement of μ-opioid receptors in antinociceptive action of botulinum toxin type A. *Neuropharmacology* **2013**, *70*, 331–337. [CrossRef]
20. Drinovac, V.; Bach-Rojecky, L.; Lacković, Z. Association of antinociceptive action of botulinum toxin type A with GABA-A receptor. *J. Neural Transm.* **2014**, *121*, 665–669. [CrossRef] [PubMed]
21. Mika, J.; Rojewska, E.; Makuch, W.; Korostynski, M.; Luvisetto, S.; Marinelli, S.; Pavone, F.; Przewlocka, B. The effect of botulinum neurotoxin A on sciatic nerve injury-induced neuroimmunological changes in rat dorsal root ganglia and spinal cord. *Neuroscience* **2011**, *175*, 358–366. [CrossRef] [PubMed]
22. Muñoz-Lora, V.R.M.; Abdalla, H.B.; Cury, A.A.D.B.; Clemente-Napimoga, J.T. Modulatory effect of botulinum toxin type A on the microglial P2X7/CatS/FKN activated-pathway in antigen-induced arthritis of the temporomandibular joint of rats. *Toxicon* **2020**, *187*, 116–121. [CrossRef] [PubMed]
23. Kurtoglu, C.; Gur, O.H.; Kurkcu, M.; Sertdemir, Y.; Guler-Uysal, F.; Uysal, H. Effect of botulinum toxin-A in myofascial pain patients with or without functional disc displacement. *J. Oral Maxillofac. Surg.* **2008**, *66*, 1644–1651. [CrossRef]
24. Ernberg, M.; Hedenberg-Magnusson, B.; List, T.; Svensson, P. Efficacy of botulinum toxin type A for treatment of persistent myofascial TMD pain: A randomized, controlled, double-blind multicenter study. *Pain* **2011**, *152*, 1988–1996. [CrossRef] [PubMed]
25. Guarda-Nardini, L.; Stecco, A.; Stecco, C.; Masiero, S.; Manfredini, D. Myofascial pain of the jaw muscles: Comparison of short-term effectiveness of botulinum toxin injections and fascial manipulation technique. *CRANIO®* **2012**, *30*, 95–102. [CrossRef] [PubMed]
26. Patel, A.A.; Lerner, M.Z.; Blitzer, A. IncobotulinumtoxinA injection for temporomandibular joint disorder: A randomized controlled pilot study. *Ann. Otol. Rhinol. Laryngol.* **2017**, *126*, 328–333. [CrossRef]
27. De la Torre Canales, G.; Poluha, R.L.; Lora, V.M.; Araújo Oliveira Ferreira, D.M.; Stuginski-Barbosa, J.; Bonjardim, L.R.; Cury, A.A.D.B.; Conti, P.C.R. Botulinum toxin type A applications for masticatory myofascial pain and trigeminal neuralgia: What is the evidence regarding adverse effects? *Clin. Oral Investig.* **2019**, *23*, 3411–3421. [CrossRef] [PubMed]
28. Montes-Carmona, J.-F.; Gonzalez-Perez, L.-M.; Infante-Cossio, P. Treatment of localized and referred masticatory myofascial pain with botulinum toxin injection. *Toxins* **2020**, *13*, 6. [CrossRef]
29. De la Torre Canales, G.; Poluha, R.L.; Pinzón, N.A.; Da Silva, B.R.; Almeida, A.M.; Ernberg, M.; Manso, A.C.; Bonjardim, L.R.; Rizzatti-Barbosa, C.M. Efficacy of botulinum toxin type-A I in the improvement of mandibular motion and muscle sensibility in myofascial pain TMD Subjects: A randomized controlled trial. *Toxins* **2022**, *14*, 441. [CrossRef]
30. Bach-Rojecky, L.; Šalković-Petrišić, M.; Lacković, Z. Botulinum toxin type A reduces pain supersensitivity in experimental diabetic neuropathy: Bilateral effect after unilateral injection. *Eur. J. Pharmacol.* **2010**, *633*, 10–14. [CrossRef]
31. Niddam, D.M. Brain manifestation and modulation of pain from myofascial trigger points. *Curr. Pain Headache Rep.* **2009**, *13*, 370–375. [CrossRef] [PubMed]
32. Tsai, C.; Lin, Y.; Su, B.; Yang, L.; Chiu, W. Masseter muscle fibre changes following reduction of masticatory function. *Int. J. Oral Maxillofac. Surg.* **2012**, *41*, 394–399. [CrossRef]
33. Balanta-Melo, J.; Toro-Ibacache, V.; Torres-Quintana, M.A.; Kupczik, K.; Vega, C.; Morales, C.; Hernández-Moya, N.; Arias-Calderón, M.; Beato, C.; Buvinic, S. Early molecular response and microanatomical changes in the masseter muscle and mandibular head after botulinum toxin intervention in adult mice. *Ann. Anat. -Anat. Anz.* **2018**, *216*, 112–119. [CrossRef]
34. Dressler, D.; Saberi, F.A. Botulinum toxin: Mechanisms of action. *Eur. Neurol.* **2005**, *53*, 3–9. [CrossRef]
35. Fortuna, R.; Vaz, M.A.; Youssef, A.R.; Longino, D.; Herzog, W. Changes in contractile properties of muscles receiving repeat injections of botulinum toxin (Botox). *J. Biomech.* **2011**, *44*, 39–44. [CrossRef]
36. Rauso, R.; Lo Giudice, G.; Tartaro, G.; Zerbinati, N.; Nicoletti, G.F.; Fragola, R. Botulinum toxin type A injections for masticatory muscles hypertrophy: A systematic review. *J. Cranio-Maxillo-Facial Surg.: Off. Publ. Eur. Assoc. Cranio-Maxillo-Facial Surg.* **2022**, *50*, 7–18. [CrossRef] [PubMed]
37. Shome, D.; Khare, S.; Kapoor, R. Efficacy of botulinum toxin in treating Asian Indian patients with masseter hypertrophy: A 4-year follow-up study. *Plast. Reconstr. Surg.* **2019**, *144*, 390e–396e. [CrossRef] [PubMed]
38. LeResche, L.; Von Korff, M. Research diagnostic criteria for temporomandibular disorders: Review, criteria, examinations and specifications, critique. *J. Craniomandib. Disord.* **1992**, *6*, 301–355.
39. Ferreira-Valente, M.A.; Pais-Ribeiro, J.L.; Jensen, M.P. Validity of four pain intensity rating scales. *Pain®* **2011**, *152*, 2399–2404. [CrossRef]
40. Isselée, H.; De Laat, A.; Bogaerts, K.; Lysens, R. Short-term reproducibility of pressure pain thresholds in masticatory muscles measured with a new algometer. *J. Orofac. Pain* **1998**, *12*, 203–209.
41. Castelo, P.M.; Duarte Gavião, M.B.; Pereira, L.J.; Bonjardim, L.R. Evaluation of changes in muscle thickness, bite force and facial asymmetry during early treatment of functional posterior crossbite. *J. Clin. Pediatr. Dent.* **2010**, *34*, 369–374. [CrossRef] [PubMed]

toxins

MDPI

Article

Effects of Botulinum Toxin Therapy on Health-Related Quality of Life Evaluated by the Oromandibular Dystonia Rating Scale

Kazuya Yoshida

Department of Oral and Maxillofacial Surgery, National Hospital Organization, Kyoto Medical Center 1-1 Mukaihata-cho, Fukakusa, Fushimi-ku, Kyoto 612-8555, Japan; yoshida.kazuya.ut@mail.hosp.go.jp; Tel.: +81-75-641-9161; Fax: +81-75-643-4325

Abstract: Oromandibular dystonia (OMD) refers to a focal dystonia in the stomatognathic system. Health-related quality of life (HRQoL) in isolated dystonia is associated with non-motor symptoms such as depression, anxiety, and pain, as well as motor symptoms. To evaluate HRQoL in patients with OMD, the therapeutic effects of botulinum neurotoxin (BoNT) therapy were assessed using a recently developed and validated comprehensive measurement tool called the Oromandibular Dystonia Rating Scale (OMDRS). Altogether, 408 patients (jaw closing dystonia, $n = 223$; tongue (lingual) dystonia, $n = 86$; jaw opening dystonia, $n = 50$; jaw deviation dystonia, $n = 23$; jaw protrusion dystonia, $n = 13$; and lip (labial) dystonia, $n = 13$) were evaluated at baseline and after the end of BoNT therapy or in a stable status. The total OMDRS score reduced significantly from 149.1 to 57.6 ($p < 0.001$). Mean improvement was 63.1%. All examiner-rated subscales (severity, disability, and pain) and patient-rated questionnaire scores (general, eating, speech, cosmetic, social/family life, sleep, annoyance, mood, and psychosocial function) were significantly lower at the endpoint than at baseline ($p < 0.001$). The BoNT injection had a highly positive impact on patient HRQoL, and the OMDRS could evaluate both motor phenomena and non-motor symptoms.

Keywords: botulinum toxin therapy; oromandibular dystonia; botulinum neurotoxin; Oromandibular Dystonia Rating Scale (OMDRS); health-related quality of life; non-motor symptom; motor symptom; jaw closing dystonia; tongue dystonia

Key Contribution: BoNT injection has a positive impact on patients with OMD. The OMDRS can be sensitive and reflective of the comprehensive evaluation of both motor and non-motor symptoms in patients with OMD as well as HRQoL and post-treatment changes with BoNT therapy.

Citation: Yoshida, K. Effects of Botulinum Toxin Therapy on Health-Related Quality of Life Evaluated by the Oromandibular Dystonia Rating Scale. *Toxins* **2022**, *14*, 656. https://doi.org/10.3390/toxins14100656

Received: 27 August 2022
Accepted: 20 September 2022
Published: 22 September 2022

1. Introduction

Dystonia is characterized by sustained or intermittent muscle contractions that cause abnormal movements or postures [1]. Oromandibular dystonia (OMD) is a focal dystonia involving the masticatory, lingual, and/or muscles in the stomatognathic system [2–14]. Based on the direction of abnormal dystonic movements, OMD is classified into six subtypes: jaw closing, jaw opening, tongue (lingual), jaw deviation, jaw protrusion, and lip (labial) dystonia [9,11–14]. Various combinations of these subtypes have been observed in several cases. A previously reported estimated prevalence of OMD varied from 0.1 to 9.8 per 100,000 persons [11,15,16]. Symptoms related to OMD include masticatory disturbances, limited mouth opening, muscle pain, dysphagia, dysarthria, esthetic problems, and temporomandibular joint dislocation [2–14]. Some patients exhibit life-threatening features, such as upper airway obstruction due to temporomandibular joint dislocation resulting from severe jaw opening dystonia [17,18] or aspiration pneumonia related to lingual dystonia [19]. These symptoms can result in impaired activities of daily living, social embarrassment, cosmetic disfigurement, absenteeism, unemployment, and a significant impact on a patient's overall HRQoL [9,13,14]. The symptoms and clinical features may be significantly more variable, critical, and complicated than those accompanied by other focal dystonia, including cervical dystonia or blepharospasm [9]. In 2002, a clinical scoring system for OMD according to subscores for pain, mastication, speech, and discomfort was reported and evaluated in 44 patients with OMD before and after muscle afferent block therapy [2,20]. In 2010, Merz et al. [21] developed and validated the Oromandibular Dystonia Questionnaire (OMDQ-25). In 2019, an oromandibular dystonia screening questionnaire was developed and validated for the differential diagnosis of OMD from other diseases such as temporomandibular disorders, dyskinesia, and functional movement disorders [8]. In 2020, a comprehensive disease-specific Oromandibular Dystonia Rating Scale (OMDRS) was developed and validated [9] (Figure S1). Although several measurement instruments have been used to evaluate various types of dystonia, only a few have been assessed in the clinimetric context [22,23].

Intramuscular injection of botulinum toxin (BoNT) has been successfully applied for OMD as a standard treatment [3–7,10,12–14]. Some researchers have attempted to assess the HRQoL in patients with OMD after BoNT therapy [24–27]. Unfortunately, the number of participants was relatively low, and differences in OMD subtypes were not considered; thus, the reliability remains uncertain. Apart from motor phenomena, there are other non-motor symptoms such as depression, anxiety, sleep problems, and pain in many patients with dystonia [28–32]. Non-motor symptoms are increasingly recognized as important determinants of HRQoL in cervical dystonia [29–32]. The objective of the present study was to evaluate post-treatment changes in BoNT therapy at the endpoint or in a stable status, particularly in the HRQoL, in patients with OMD using the OMDRS.

2. Results

2.1. Demographic Data and Results of Treatment

The demographic characteristics of 408 patients (262 women, 146 men; mean age 52.0 ± 15.6 years (standard deviation [SD])) with OMD are summarized in Table 1. Women (53.8 ± 15.9 years) were significantly ($p < 0.005$, unpaired t-test) older than men (48.7 ± 14.4 years). One hundred sixty-eight patients (41.2%) had tardive dystonia. Seventy-three patients (17.9%) had other types of dystonia such as cervical dystonia (10.5%) or blepharospasm (6.1%) (Table 1). However, the symptoms of these types of dystonia were very mild, and the chief complaints were symptoms associated with OMD.

Table 1. Demographic characteristics for each subtype of OMD.

Subtypes	Jaw Closing	Tongue	Jaw Opening	Jaw Deviation	Jaw Protrusion	Lip	Total
No. of patients [N]	223	86	50	23	13	13	408
Age (years) [mean (SD)] (range)	53.8 (15.6) (18–95)	48.3 (14.3) (24–86)	52.3 (18.1) (19–86)	51.5 (15.7) (26–81)	49.2 (11.4) (21–63)	48.7 (11.8) (37–68)	52.0 (15.6) (18–95)
Sex (women, men) [N (%)]	155 (69.5), 68(30.5)	51 (59.3), 35 (40.7)	26 (51.0), 24 (47.1)	14 (60.9), 9 (39.1)	7 (53.8), 6 (46.2)	10 (76.9), 3 (23.1)	262 (64.2), 146 (35.8)
Duration (months) [mean (SD)] (range)	51.5 (64.6) (1–276)	39.0 (68.5) (1–180)	48.7 (91.5) (1–180)	41.0 (52.3) (2–228)	26.0 (22.1) (3–60)	56.8 (47.3) (4–156)	47.3 (67.3) (1–276)
Tardive dystonia [N (%)]	101 (45.3)	27 (31.4)	23 (45.1)	7 (30.4)	4 (28.6)	6 (46.2)	168 (41.2)
Other dystonia [N (%)]	41 (18.4)	7 (8.1)	17 (34.0)	4 (17.4)	1 (7.7)	3 (23.1)	73 (17.9)
Cervical dystonia	28 (12.6)	1 (1.2)	9 (18.0)	2 (8.7)	1 (7.7)	2 (15.4)	43 (10.5)
Blepharospasm	16 (7.2)	2 (2.3)	4 (8.0)	2 (8.7)	0	1 (7.7)	25 (6.1)
Writer's cramp	3 (1.3)	2 (2.3)	2 (4.0)	0	0	0	7 (1.7)
Upper limb dystonia	2 (0.9)	1 (1.2)	1 (2.0)	1 (4.3)	0	0	5 (1.2)
Lower limb dystonia	2 (0.9)	0	1 (2.0)	0	0	0	3 (0.7)
Spasmodic dysphonia	1 (0.4)	0	1 (2.0)	0	0	1 (7.7)	3 (0.7)
Embouchure dystonia	1 (0.4)	1 (1.2)	0	0	0	0	2 (0.5)

The main symptoms of the patients were masticatory disturbance (n = 146, 35.8%), discomfort, cosmetic problems associated with involuntary movement (n = 123, 30.1%), pain ($n = 78$, 19.1%), dysarthria ($n = 68$, 16.7%), and dysphagia ($n = 41$, 10.0%). Evaluation of the OMDRS revealed that such symptoms were more prevalent (cosmetic problem ($n = 314$, 77.0%), masticatory disturbance ($n = 267$, 65.2%), dysarthria ($n = 230$, 56.4%), pain ($n = 199$, 48.8%), and dysphagia ($n = 159$, 38.9%)).

The results of BoNT therapy are shown in Table 2. The mean number of BoNT injection was 5.4 ± 5.0. The main target muscles were the masseter (86.1%), temporalis (49.3%), and medial pterygoid muscles (17.5%) for jaw closing dystonia; the genioglossus and other tongue muscles (100%) and lateral pterygoid muscle (22.1%) for tongue dystonia; the lateral pterygoid muscle (96–100%) for jaw opening, jaw deviation, and jaw protrusion dystonia; and the orbicularis oris (69.2%), risorius (61.5%), and mentalis muscles (38.5%) for lip dystonia (Table 2). The mean number of injected muscles was 3.7 ± 2.0 (Table 2). There were no significant differences in the mean number of injections or injected muscles among the subtypes of OMD.

Table 2. Results of BoNT injection for each subtype of OMD.

	Jaw Closing	Tongue	Jaw Opening	Jaw Deviation	Jaw Protrusion	Lip	Total
No. of patients [N]	223	86	50	23	13	13	408
No. of BoNT injection [mean (SD)], (range)	4.7 (4.4) (2–22)	6.4 (5.6) (3–27)	6.1 (5.2) (2–25)	6.4 (6.1) (3–25)	4.2 (3.1) (2–9)	5.8 (5.7) (2–17)	5.4 (5.0) (2–27)
No. of injected muscles [mean (SD)], (range)	3.9 (1.9) (1–12)	3.1 (1.8) (2–12)	3.8 (2.2) (2–10)	3.8 (2.4) (1–6)	3.3 (1.7) (2–6)	4.4 (1.9) (1–8)	3.7 (2.0) (1–12)
Target muscles [N (%)]	Masseter: 192 (86.1) Temporalis: 110 (49.3) Medial pterygoid: 39 (17.5) Lateral pterygoid: 26 (11.7) Posterior digastric: 10 (4.5) Orbicularis oris: 8 (3.6) Mentalis: 8 (3.6) Genioglossus: 8 (3.6) Sternocleidomastoid: 6 (2.7) Risorius: 5 (2.2) Zygomatic major 3 (1.3) Others: 7 (3.1)	Genioglossus: 86 (100) Lateral pterygoid: 19 (22.1) Masseter: 10 (11.6) Medial pterygoid: 3 (3.5) Orbicularis oris 3 (3.5) Temporalis: 2 (2.3) Posterior digastric: 2 (2.3) Others: 3 (3.5)	Lateral pterygoid: 48 (96) Anterior digastric: 10 (20) Posterior digastric: 8 (16) Genioglossus: 7 (14) Orbicularis oris 3 (6) Sternocleidomastoid: 3 (6) Platysma: 3 (6) Mentalis: 2 (4) Risorius: 1 (2)	Lateral pterygoid: 23 (100) Masseter: 7 (30.4) Temporalis: 4 (17.4) Risorius: 3 (13) Posterior digastric: 2 (9.5) Others: 4 (13)	Lateral pterygoid: 13 (100) Masseter: 3 (23.1) Temporalis: 3 (23.1)	Orbicularis oris: 9 (69.2) Risorius: 8 (61.5) Mentalis: 5 (38.5) Depressor labii inferioris: 3 (23.1) Masseter: 2 (15.4) Others: 3 (23.1)	Masseter: 210 (51.5) Lateral pterygoid: 129 (31.6) Temporalis: 119 (29.2) Genioglossus: 101 (24.8) Medical pterygoid: 42 (10.3) Orbicularis oris: 23 (5.6) Posterior digastric: 22 (5.4) Risorius: 17 (4.2) Mentalis: 15 (3.7)Anterior digastric: 10 (2.5) Sternocleidomastoid: 9 (2.2) Zygomatic major 3 (0.7) Platysma: 3 (0.7) Depressor labii inferioris: 3 (0.7) Others: 17 (4.2)
Improvement (%) [mean (SD)], (range)	63.3 (16.2) 17.1–98.1	66.3 (20.8) 21.4–97.8	57.2 (23.1) 14.9–98.4	65.8 (19.2) 28.7–87.1	58.8 (17.5) 35.0–80.5	60.6 (15.1) 31.9–86.6	63.1 (18.6) 14.9–98.4
Partial responder [N (%)]	3 (1.3)	4 (4.7)	6 (12.0)	1 (4.3)	0	0	14 (3.4)
Follow-up (months) [mean (SD)], (range)	27.8 (22.9) (12–98)	37.2 (29.3) (12–87)	35.6 (27.9) (12–74)	38.4 (34.9) (12–78)	23.6 (17.9) (12–32)	38.1 (37.1) (12–62)	31.8 (28.8) (12–87)

The mean improvement in the total OMDRS scores was 63.1 ± 18.6%. Fourteen patients (jaw closing, $n = 3$; tongue, $n = 4$; jaw opening, $n = 6$; and jaw deviation, $n = 1$) qualified as partial responders (<30% improvement in total OMDRS score). The proportion of partial responders was significantly higher in jaw opening dystonia (6/50 patients) than in jaw closing dystonia (3/223 patients; $p < 0.005$, Fisher's exact test). Ten (71.4%) of the 14 partial responders had tardive dystonia, and five patients had other dystonia (cervical dystonia, $n = 4$ and blepharospasm, $n = 1$). The mean follow-up duration from the first visit to the evaluation using the OMDRS for this study was 31.8 ± 28.8 months (Table 2). There were no significant differences in the mean improvement and follow-up among the subtypes of OMD.

Pain scores at baseline were significantly higher in women (10.5 ± 10.8) than in men (6.9 ± 9.5; $p < 0.005$). Examiner-rated scores were also significantly higher in women (27.0 ± 14.7) than in men (23.7 ± 12.7; $p < 0.005$). At the endpoint, women (3.9 ± 5.4) showed significantly higher pain scores than men (2.0 ± 3.5; $p < 0.005$), and significantly higher scores in sleep than men (2.7 ± 3.7 vs. 1.8 ± 2.5; $p < 0.05$).

The adverse effects were temporary regional weakness and tenderness at the injection sites. Approximately 10% of patients with lingual dystonia had mild or transient difficulty in swallowing. Adverse unfavorable events were transient and spontaneously disappeared within 1–2 weeks. No other significant complications were noted.

2.2. OMDRS Scores at Baseline and Endpoint

The results of the OMDRS scores (Figure S1) at the baseline and endpoint are summarized in Table 3. Examiner-rated subscales (severity, disability (activities of daily living), and pain) were significantly higher in jaw closing dystonia (27.6 ± 14.3) than in tongue dystonia (21.4 ± 12.3; $p < 0.01$) (Figure 1). Patient-rated questionnaire scores (general, eating, speech, cosmetic, social/family life, sleep, annoyance, mood, and psychosocial function) were significantly higher in jaw opening dystonia (144.1 ± 56.5) than in jaw closing dystonia (115.9 ± 55.0; $p < 0.01$) (Figure 1). OMDRS scores were significantly higher in jaw opening dystonia (170.5 ± 64.1) than in jaw closing dystonia (115.9 ± 62.4; $p < 0.05$) (Figure 1). At the endpoint, patient-rated scores were significantly higher in jaw opening dystonia (65.6 ± 41.8) than in jaw closing dystonia (42.1 ± 29.7; $p < 0.05$) (Figure 1).

Table 3. OMDRS scores at baseline and endpoint.

OMDRS Subscale (Range)	Baseline	Endpoint	*p*-Value
Examiner-rated scale [mean (SD)]			
Severity (0–16)	7.5 (2.9)	3.3 (2.4)	$p < 0.001$
Disability (0–30)	9.1 (5.6)	3.6 (3.9)	$p < 0.001$
Pain (0–40)	9.3 (10.6)	3.2 (4.8)	$p < 0.001$
Total examiner-rated scores (0–86)	25.9 (14.1)	10.0 (9.1)	$p < 0.001$
Patient-rated questionnaire [mean (SD)]			
General (0–20)	14.2 (4.4)	5.7 (3.7)	$p < 0.001$
Eating (0–28)	10.3 (7.7)	4.4 (4.6)	$p < 0.001$
Speech (0–16)	8.0 (5.0)	3.3 (3.1)	$p < 0.001$
Cosmetic (0–28)	12.8 (8.0)	4.6 (4.6)	$p < 0.001$
Social/family life (0–20)	8.8 (5.7)	4.3 (4.1)	$p < 0.001$
Sleep (0–16)	5.1 (5.3)	2.4 (3.2)	$p < 0.001$
Annoyance (0–32)	16.2 (7.8)	7.8 (6.6)	$p < 0.001$
Mood (0–28)	16.2 (7.8)	8.3 (6.4)	$p < 0.001$
Psychosocial functioning (0–40)	15.0 (10.5)	8.0 (7.5)	$p < 0.001$
Total patient-rated scores (0–228)	123.9 (53.2)	48.2 (34.8)	$p < 0.001$
OMDRS (0–314)	148.9 (59.6)	57.6 (40.6)	$p < 0.001$

Improvement, calculated as the rate of decrease in the total OMDRS score, was significantly correlated ($r = 0.938$; $p < 0.001$) with subjective improvement. Post-treatment OMDRS scores showed a significant correlation ($r = 0.231$; $p < 0.005$) with the number of injected muscles and were significantly negatively correlated ($r = -0.302$; $p < 0.001$) with improvement in OMDRS scores.

The total OMDRS score reduced significantly from 149.1 ± 71.3 to 57.6 ± 40.6 ($p < 0.001$) (Table 3). All examiner-rated subscales (severity, disability, and pain) and patient-rated questionnaires (general, eating, speech, cosmetic, social/family life, sleep, annoyance, mood, and psychosocial functioning) showed significantly lower scores after BoNT therapy ($p < 0.001$) (Table 3).

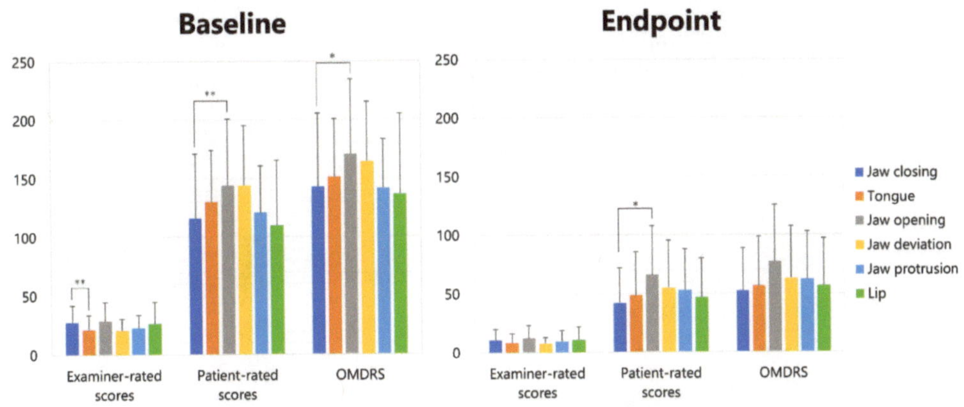

Figure 1. Scores of examiner-rated scale and patient-rated questionnaire scores of each subtype of OMD at baseline and endpoint. * $p < 0.05$, ** $p < 0.01$.

2.3. Differences in Subscales Scores of OMDRS among Subtypes of OMD

Scores of each subscale in each subtype of OMD are shown in Figure 2 (at baseline) and Figure 3 (at the endpoint).

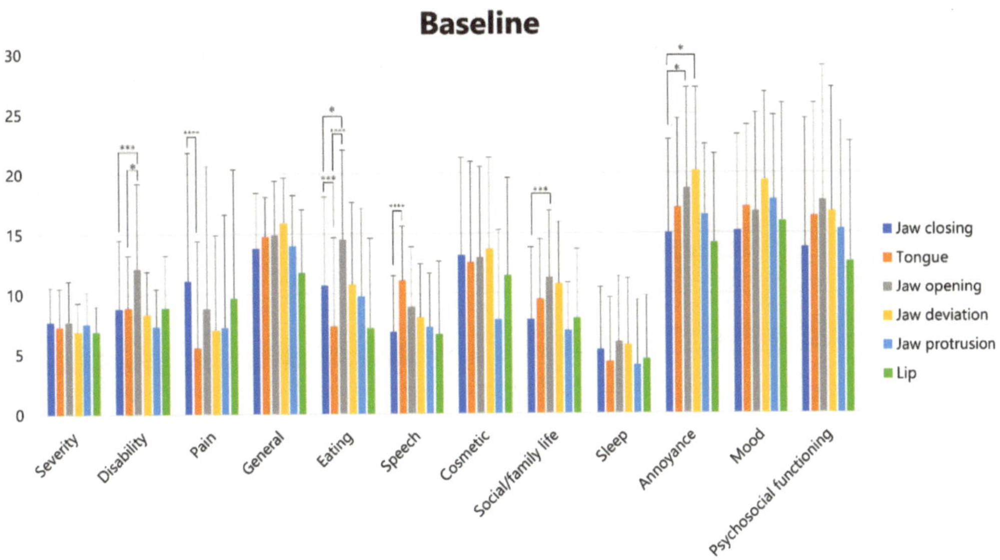

Figure 2. Scores of subscales of OMDRS in each subtype of OMD at baseline. * $p < 0.05$, *** $p < 0.005$, **** $p < 0.001$.

At baseline, one-way analysis of variance revealed significant differences in disability, pain, eating, speech, social/family life, and annoyance (Figure 2). The disability scores of jaw opening dystonia (12.1 ± 7.1) were significantly higher than those of jaw closing dystonia (8.8 ± 5.7; $p < 0.005$) and tongue dystonia (8.9 ± 4.3; $p < 0.05$). Pain scores of jaw closing dystonia (11.1 ± 10.7) were significantly higher than those of tongue dystonia (5.5 ± 8.9; $p < 0.001$). The eating scores of tongue dystonia (7.3 ± 7.4) were significantly lower than those of jaw opening dystonia (14.5 ± 7.5, $p < 0.001$) and jaw closing dystonia (10.7 ± 7.4, $p < 0.001$), and the eating scores of jaw opening dystonia (14.5 ± 7.5) were significantly higher than those of jaw closing dystonia (10.7 ± 7.4, $p < 0.05$). The speech scores of tongue dystonia (11.1 ± 4.5) were significantly higher than those of jaw closing dystonia (6.8 ± 4.7; $p < 0.001$). The social/family life scores of jaw opening dystonia (11.3 ± 5.6) were significantly higher than those of jaw closing dystonia (7.8 ± 6.0; $p < 0.005$). Annoyance scores of jaw opening (17.7 ± 11.2) were significantly higher than those of jaw closing dystonia (13.8 ± 10.7; $p < 0.05$) and tongue dystonia (16.4 ± 9.4; $p < 0.05$).

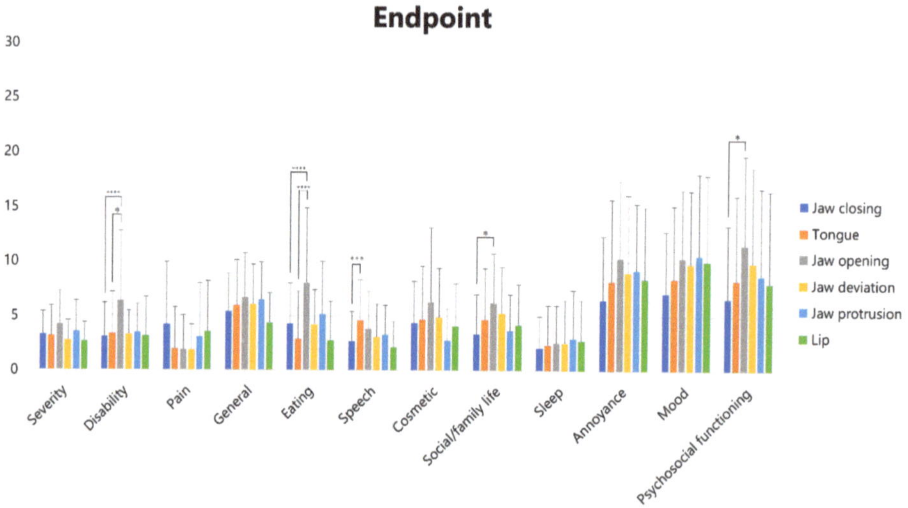

Figure 3. Scores of subscales of OMDRS in each subtype of OMD at the endpoint. * $p < 0.05$, *** $p < 0.005$, **** $p < 0.001$.

At the endpoint, one-way analysis of variance revealed significant differences in disability, eating, speech, social/family life, and psychosocial functioning (Figure 3).

The disability scores of jaw opening dystonia (6.4 ± 6.4) were significantly higher than those of jaw closing dystonia (3.1 ± 3.1, $p < 0.001$) and tongue dystonia (3.4 ± 3.8, $p < 0.05$). The eating scores of jaw opening dystonia (8.0 ± 6.9) were significantly higher than those of tongue dystonia (2.9 ± 4.4; $p < 0.001$) and jaw closing dystonia (4.3 ± 3.7; $p < 0.001$). The speech scores of tongue dystonia (4.6 ± 3.7) were significantly higher than those of jaw closing dystonia (2.7 ± 2.7; $p < 0.005$). Scores of social/family life of jaw opening dystonia (6.2 ± 4.5) were significantly higher than those of jaw closing dystonia (3.4 ± 3.6; $p < 0.05$). The psychosocial functioning scores of jaw opening (11.5 ± 8.2) were significantly higher than those of jaw closing dystonia (6.6 ± 6.7; $p < 0.05$) and tongue dystonia (16.4 ± 9.4; $p < 0.05$).

2.4. *Differences in OMDRS Scores between Idiopathic and Tardive Cases*

The total OMDRS scores at baseline were significantly higher in patients with tardive dystonia (172.1 ± 69.6) than in idiopathic patients (132.3 ± 54.1; $p < 0.001$, unpaired *t*-test). The OMDRS scores at the endpoint also showed significant differences (74.9 ± 41.4 vs. 46.8 ± 36.2, $p < 0.005$). The improvement was significantly lower in tardive cases (58.7 ± 17.8%) than in idiopathic cases (65.9 ± 18.6%; $p < 0.001$). Subjective improvement was also significantly lower in tardive patients (52.3 ± 18.8%) than in idiopathic patients (67.6 ± 17.4%, $p < 0.001$). Improvements in patient-rated scores were significantly lower in tardive patients (57.4 ± 17.8%) than in idiopathic patients (65.5 ± 19.1%, $p < 0.001$).

Although improvement of examiner-rated score was lower in tardive cases (60.6 ± 20.1%) than in idiopathic cases (64.6 ± 20.3%), it was not significant ($p = 0.15$).

Most scores of the subscales of the OMDRS were significantly higher (unpaired t-test) in patients with tardive dystonia than in those with idiopathic dystonia (Figure 4). At baseline, significant differences were observed in severity (7.9 ± 3.1 vs. 7.3 ± 2.8, $p < 0.05$), disability (10.8 ± 5.7 vs. 7.9 ± 5.2, $p < 0.001$), general (15.1 ± 4.5 vs. 13.6 ± 4.2, $p < 0.001$), eating (12.6 ± 7.3 vs. 8.6 ± 7.5, $p < 0.001$), social/family life (10.9 ± 5.8 vs. 7.2 ± 5.2, $p < 0.001$), sleep (6.4 ± 5.5 vs. 4.1 ± 4.9, $p < 0.001$), annoyance (18.7 ± 7.7 vs. 14.6 ± 7.6, $p < 0.001$), mood (± vs. ±, $p < 0.001$), and psychosocial functioning (19.0 ± 11.0 vs. 12.1 ± 9.1, $p < 0.001$) (Figure 4). At the endpoint, significant differences were observed in disability (4.5 ± 3.8 vs. 3.1 ± 3.8, $p < 0.01$), general (6.5 ± 3.9 vs. 5.3 ± 3.5, $p < 0.05$), social/family life (6.4 ± 4.3 vs. 2.9 ± 3.4, $p < 0.001$), sleep (3.7 ± 3.9 vs. 1.5 ± 2.5, $p < 0.001$), annoyance (11.3 ± 6.8 vs. 5.6 ± 5.4, $p < 0.001$), mood (11.6 ± 6.7 vs. 6.3 ± 5.2, $p < 0.001$), and psychosocial functioning (11.8 ± 7.8 vs. 5.6 ± 6.2, $p < 0.001$) (Figure 4).

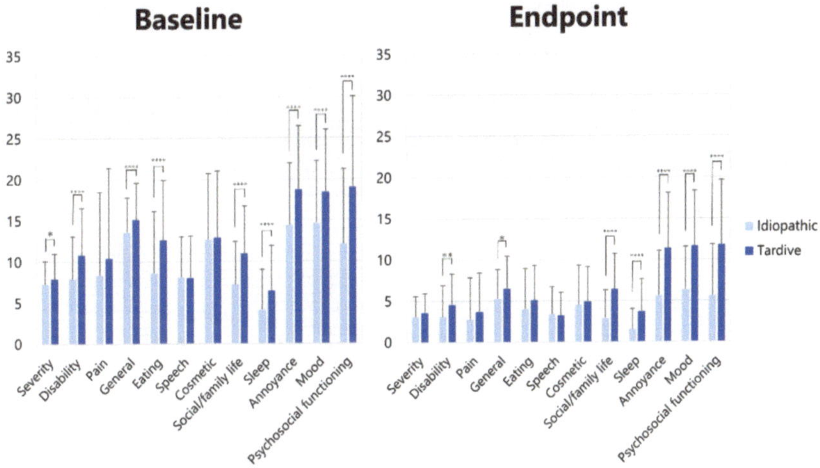

Figure 4. Scores of subscales of OMDRS in idiopathic and tardive cases at baseline and endpoint. * $p < 0.05$, ** $p < 0.01$, **** $p < 0.001$.

3. Discussion

This study is the first to report therapeutic effects and post-treatment changes in HRQoL in patients with OMD after BoNT therapy using a comprehensive measurement tool. Differences were compared among the six OMD subtypes in the present study. The OMDRS precisely assessed motor and non-motor features after BoNT therapy, even for each subtype of OMD. Jaw opening dystonia tended to be more severe in disability, eating, and social family/life; jaw closing in pain; and tongue dystonia was severe in speech.

3.1. Rating Scales for OMD

Merz et al. [21] developed and validated the OMDQ-25, which consists of five subscales (general, psychosocial, cosmesis, speech, and eating dysfunction). This scale was the first measurement tool to assess the HRQoL in patients with OMD. However, the Movement Disorders Society Task Force on dystonia rating scales did not recommend the OMDQ-25 but merely suggested it because it was used only by the original developers and not by other researchers [22]. Subsequently, the OMDQ-25 was applied in several studies [9,33,34]. OMD symptoms exhibit extremely large individual differences among patients. For instance, jaw closing, jaw opening, and tongue dystonia are completely different in terms of clinical features, affected muscles with abnormal contracture, and direction of abnormal movements. Therefore, the severity subscale should be examined according to OMD subtype. However, if the items are negatively associated within a subscale, the subscale cannot reach sufficient internal consistency, as assessed by Cronbach's alpha [35]. Therefore, in the OMDRS, only the severity subscale (four items) was assigned five patterns according to the OMD subtype (jaw closing, tongue, jaw opening, jaw deviation (protrusion), and lip dystonia) [9]. The OMDQ-25 is a concise, patient-rated 25-item questionnaire [21]. In contrast, the OMDRS includes a 15-item examiner-rated scale and a 57-item patient-administered questionnaire to comprehensively assess the full spectrum of OMD [9]. Significant correlations between the subscales of the OMDRS and the Short Form-36 Health Survey were reported for several subscales (pain, general, eating, social/family life, sleep, annoyance, and psychosocial functioning) [9]. The OMDRS can be useful for more precise evaluation of disease severity and post-treatment changes in each subtype for both clinical and research purposes.

The patient-administered rating scale, particularly the Cervical Dystonia Impact Profile-58 [36], is more sensitive and reflective of HRQoL than the physician-administered standard recommended measure of cervical dystonia severity in patients after BoNT injection [30]. Four subscales (sleep, annoyance, mood, and psychosocial functioning), a disease-specific questionnaire, and an examiner-rated scale were combined to construct the OMDRS [9] (Figure S1). Therefore, the OMDRS can be sensitive and reflective of non-motor symptoms and health-related quality of life in OMD, as can the Cervical Dystonia Impact Profile-58 in cervical dystonia. Non-motor symptoms are highly prevalent in cervical dystonia [29–32]. Non-motor symptoms are increasingly recognized as important determinants of HRQoL in various movement disorders [28–32]. Motor improvement after BoNT therapy for cervical dystonia did not correlate with non-motor changes [32]. In BoNT therapy for OMD, special attention should be paid not only to the motor symptoms but also to the non-motor symptoms in order to improve the patient's HRQoL.

The chief complaints of the patients (masticatory disturbance, 35.8%; discomfort and cosmetic problems associated with involuntary movement, 30.1%; pain, 19.1%; dysarthria, 16.7%; and dysphagia, 10.0%) were more prevalent (cosmetic problems, 77.0%; masticatory disturbance, 65.2%; dysarthria, 56.4%; pain, 48.8%; and dysphagia, 38.9%) after evaluation of OMDRS. The OMDRS could be used to evaluate very mild symptoms other than the chief complaint in more detail.

3.2. *Results of This Study*

This study was based on real-world clinical results obtained by an OMD specialist. The author has treated several thousands of patients with a variety of movement disorders in the stomatognathic system over the past 30 years. Moreover, the author was able to clinically and scientifically research movement disorders with many neurologists. In the present study, the improvement evaluated by the reduction rate of OMDRS scores was 63.1% without significant adverse effects. Merz et al. [21] reported a reduction rate of 37.6%, Nastasi et al. [33] 15.4%, and Scorr et al. [34] 19.8%, as recalculated by the percentage reduction of the OMDQ-25. The much higher success rate without complications in this study than that of previous studies may be related to the following factors. First, oral surgeons must be more familiar with masticatory and other muscles in the stomatognathic system than neurologists, otorhinolaryngologists, and other medical professionals. A complete understanding of the local anatomy of the stomatognathic system is a prerequisite for target muscle selection and safe injection without complications [12–14,37]. The more accurately BoNT is administered to the target muscles, the more likely is the improvement in patient symptoms, and the lower the risk of complications [12–14,37]. Second, dental problems such as temporomandibular disorders and bruxism were differentially diagnosed and excluded from BoNT therapy by an expert oral surgeon. Third, patients who were not indicated for BoNT injection, such as those with functional movement disorder [38] or psychiatric disease, were excluded using a muscle afferent block (lidocaine injection) before BoNT therapy [12–14,39].

Berardelli et al. [40] reported that dystonic movement in patients with cervical dystonia evaluated using the Toronto Torticollis Rating Scale showed significant improvement after

5 years of BoNT therapy (33.4 vs. 26.9). However, neuropsychiatric disorders did not improve at all (65% vs. 64%). Widespread loss of inhibition and pathologically increased plasticity appear to play important roles in the pathophysiology of primary dystonia [41]. Stamelou et al. [42] proposed that the non-motor symptoms of dystonia may be explained by a common pathophysiological deficit that also underlies the motor features. Fifty-one (57.3%) of eighty-nine consecutive patients with various forms of focal dystonia had psychiatric disorders, which started on average 18.4 years before the onset of dystonia, implying that psychiatric features were primary rather than consequences of the movement disorder [43]. In this study, 41.2% of patients had tardive dystonia. Patients with tardive dystonia showed significantly higher scores on the subscales of non-motor symptoms, such as social/family life, sleep, annoyance, mood, and psychosocial functioning (Figure 4). Additional psychiatric treatment may be necessary for patients with mental disorders. A number of patients in the present study lost their jobs because of symptoms related to OMD. However, several patients could return to work after BoNT therapy, and their quality of life and mental status improved considerably.

Fourteen patients were partial responders (<30% improvement in the total OMDRS score) in this study. Ten patients presented with tardive dystonia. Whether tardive dystonia or primary non-response was the reason for the partial response remains unknown. However, improvement in the patient-rated score was significantly lower in tardive patients (57.4 ± 17.8%) than in idiopathic patients (65.5 ± 19.1%, $p < 0.001$) in this study. Moreover, scores for non-motor symptoms (annoyance, mood, and psychosocial functioning) were significantly ($p < 0.001$) higher in tardive cases than in idiopathic cases (Figure 4). The differences might result in low improvement in the ten patients. The possibility of non-responders was not confirmed in laboratory or clinical tests.

The rate of partial responders was significantly higher for jaw opening dystonia than for jaw closing dystonia. A significantly lower effect of BoNT therapy in jaw opening dystonia than in jaw closing dystonia has been reported [44]. This is considered to be related to the difficulty of accurate injection into the jaw opening muscles (the lateral pterygoid muscle and anterior belly of the digastric muscle) compared to that into the jaw closing muscles (the masseter, temporalis, and medial pterygoid muscles). As the author always injects BoNT under electromyographic (EMG) guidance, BoNT must be administered precisely to the lateral pterygoid or digastric muscles. Moreover, the author used a computer-aided design/computer-assisted manufacture-derived insertion guide into the lateral pterygoid muscles for patients with jaw opening who responded insufficiently to freehand insertion [37,45]. The lateral pterygoid is a muscle involved in mastication and usually has two heads: the inferior (lower) and superior (upper) [46–48]. As the bilateral inferior heads contract, the condyle is pulled forward and slightly downward. If the muscle is activated only on one side, the inferior jaw rotates around a vertical axis that runs through the contralateral condyle and is pulled medially to the contralateral side [46–48]. The superior and inferior heads are activated alternately during chewing, such that the inferior head contracts during mouth opening, while the superior head relaxes [46–48]. Nevertheless, the number of lateral pterygoid muscle heads remains controversial. It is commonly a two-headed muscle, but one-headed or three-headed muscles have also been reported [46,49,50]. Detailed findings of the origins and insertions of an anatomical study suggest that the lateral pterygoid muscle is a single muscle with no clear border, containing fibers in various directions, indicating that a two-head muscle pattern would be indicated by the differences in the convergences of the muscle fibers [49]. In contrast, a recent systematic review reported that the frequency of one-headed lateral pterygoid muscles ranged from 7.7% to 26.7%, two-headed muscles from 61.4% to 91.1%, and three-headed muscles from 4.0% to 35.0% [50]. The difference in efficacy of BoNT therapy between jaw closing and jaw opening dystonia may be associated with the anatomical variability of the lateral pterygoid muscle. However, further studies with larger sample sizes are warranted.

Post-treatment OMDRS scores were significantly correlated with the number of injected muscles and significantly negatively correlated with improvement. In other words, the more affected the muscles, the less effective the BoNT therapy for OMD. As there was no correlation between the degree of improvement and disease duration, it is unlikely that only the exacerbation or expansion of symptoms due to long-term disease duration affected the improvement. Whether the relatively reduced dose of BoNT due to the increased number of muscles affected this improvement was not determined. Therefore, further research is necessary.

3.3. Treatment Modalities of OMD

A recent study reported the crude prevalence of OMD to be 9.8 per 100,000, suggesting that OMD may have an equal or even higher prevalence than cervical dystonia or blepharospasm [11]. Patients with OMD were referred to dentists (70%) or oral surgeons (60%) [51]. However, approximately 90% of patients had not been diagnosed with OMD, and the vast majority of patients had been diagnosed with temporomandibular disorders, bruxism, or psychiatric diseases [11,51]. OMD has been recognized as a rare disease by many neurologists; however, in reality, cases are incorrectly diagnosed [13,14].

OMD has been regarded as the most challenging dystonia for neurologists [52]. However, it can be part of the clinical spectrum of various neurological diseases, including Parkinson's disease, Wilson's disease, ischemic or hemorrhagic stroke, tumors, infarction, and brain injury [53]. If such diseases have already been diagnosed and treated, OMD must be addressed simultaneously by the attending physicians. Likewise, collaboration with a psychiatrist is required for the treatment of tardive or functional (psychogenic) dystonia [13,14]. Neurological knowledge and experience are indispensable in the diagnosis of neurological diseases. Dental knowledge and experience are required for differential diagnosis of dental and oral conditions. Since dentists and oral surgeons are specialists of the stomatognathic system, they are likely to perform more skillful and accurate injections into the muscles in the oral region than medical professionals [13,14]. Collaboration with medical and dental professionals is important for diagnosis and treatment.

Treatment of OMD must be multimodal and highly individualized for each patient. Treatment options are oral medication [53,54], BoNT [3–7,12–14,55–59], muscle afferent block [2,20,60], occlusal splint [61,62], and surgical procedure (coronoidotomy) [63–65]. BoNT therapy, namely, chemodenervation with BoNT, is considered the first-line treatment for OMD [6,13,14]. A complete understanding of the local anatomy of the muscles, nerves, and other tissues and accurate injection procedures are prerequisites for BoNT therapy of OMD [13,14,39]. It is important to differentially diagnose the indications for BoNT injections. If an adequate dose of BoNT can be correctly administered to the affected muscles, the symptoms will improve. Previously reported adverse effects of BoNT include temporary regional weakness, tenderness or pain at the injection site, minor discomfort during chewing, asymmetric smiles, muscle atrophy, paresthesia, and difficulty in swallowing [4,56,58,59]. The majority of these side effects are thought to be related to the injection technique and are avoided by accurate knowledge of the local anatomy, precise injection procedures, and optimal dose of BoNT [13,14].

The author created websites for involuntary movements, which seem to have received considerable attention from many patients with OMD [51]. A large number of patients worldwide wish to visit our department for treatment of OMD; however, only a few can actually visit because of very high costs, including airfare [51]. Furthermore, overseas travel was prohibited due to coronavirus disease 2019 restrictions, making it impossible for patients from abroad to receive medical examinations. A computer-aided design and manufacturing process was used to develop a needle guide to reliably administer BoNT to the inferior head of the lateral pterygoid muscle [45]. Computed tomography scans with a plaster cast model of the maxilla data can be transmitted over the Internet from anywhere in the world. Telemedicine for OMD using digital technology in the era of coronavirus disease 2019, computer-aided design, and manufacturing of needle guides for lateral pterygoid muscle injection can be applied in response to the demands of overseas patients with OMD [13,14,45].

3.4. Limitations and Strengths

The present study had some limitations that should be considered. An obvious limitation of this retrospective study was its open-label design without a placebo-controlled group. It is likely that the placebo effect influenced the results of this study, particularly some subscales, such as annoyance, mood, and psychosocial functioning. Another weakness of this study was the lack of assessment of depression or anxiety using a dedicated rating scale or specialized examination. Further randomized controlled studies evaluating the mental status in greater detail are necessary.

A strength of this study was that all patients were diagnosed, treated, and evaluated by an OMD specialist to ensure the uniformity of the results. Therefore, inter-clinician or inter-rater differences in diagnosis, treatment, and rating were minimal. Furthermore, because the developers of the rating scale evaluated it themselves, the errors associated with the evaluation or rating might be minimal. Another strength of this study was the number of participants. Approximately 100 patients with various movement disorders of the stomatognathic system visit our department every week. The author launched a website for involuntary movements for both patients and healthcare workers (https://sites.google.com/site/oromandibulardystoniaenglish/, accessed on 1 August 2022) in 2011 [54]. The website has 20 versions in 20 languages. This site has been accessed tens of millions of times, worldwide. Many patients who had already abandoned treatment or further consultation visited our department from all over Japan and abroad [51]. In addition, the author has published many scientific papers and lectures on OMD, not only in neurological but also in dental or maxillofacial surgical societies and patient associations. Efforts to raise awareness about OMD have resulted in an increasing number of referrals from neurologists, neurosurgeons, dentists, oral surgeons, and otorhinolaryngologists.

3.5. Future Directions

BoNT injections have been commonly used for OMD. However, the available evidence is insufficient. An early double-blind, placebo-controlled study of BoNT treatment for cranial–cervical dystonia in 10 patients with oromandibular–cervical dystonia [55] was published, and a recent pilot single-blind study evaluated BoNT dosing and efficacy in 18 patients with OMD [34]. Unfortunately, the small number of patients, low improvement, and high frequency of side effects in these studies might limit the conclusions of BoNT therapy for OMD as an effective treatment choice. However, most other studies on BoNT therapy for OMD were based on retrospective chart reviews. Meanwhile, randomized controlled trials have already been reported for bruxism or temporomandibular disorders, which have symptoms similar to jaw closing dystonia and involuntary jaw closing [66–68]. This is likely because bruxism and temporal disorders have a higher prevalence than OMD and there are many more clinicians and researchers. In future, randomized controlled trials with a higher level of evidence should be conducted for OMD.

Although BoNT is frequently used for treatment in many countries, it has not been officially approved for OMD treatment. Well-designed, randomized, controlled trials with larger sample sizes and longer follow-up periods are required to determine the therapeutic efficacy, optimal dose, duration of effect, adverse effects, brand-specific differences, and definite indications, and to establish a protocol for BoNT therapy [13]. However, the presence of disabilities in patients with OMD places constraints on the traditional placebo–control trial design [34]. The apparent lack of effect in the control group may have led to substantial dropouts and compromised the reliability of the statistical analyses. Patients seeking OMD specialists visit from very long distances with very high expectations, making the formation of a control group ethically difficult [13]. However, such randomized controlled studies are indispensable for the official approval of BoNT and evidence-based medicine. The author, along with neurologists specializing in dystonia, is currently planning a randomized, double-blind, placebo-controlled study of BoNT therapy for OMD to seek official approval for BoNT in Japan. We hope to report on evidence-based data in the near future.

A common treatment strategy for dystonia concentrates only on physical symptoms. Nevertheless, HRQoL in isolated dystonia is strongly related to non-motor symptoms and less associated with motor symptoms [31]. Very little attention has been paid to non-motor symptoms in patients with OMD. Comprehensive treatment for OMD should address both physical and mental aspects. Some patients with OMD may require additional mental health care. For this purpose, collaboration with psychiatrists may be necessary, indicating the importance of dental and medical multidisciplinary team approaches.

4. Conclusions

BoNT therapy is very effective and safe for OMD when properly diagnosed and administered precisely. The OMDRS can be used to comprehensively evaluate therapeutic effects and HRQoL.

5. Materials and Methods

5.1. Participants

Four hundred and eight patients (262 women and 146 men; mean age, 52.0 ± 15.6 years) with OMD, who visited our department from January 2016 to January 2021, were enrolled in this retrospective study (Table 1). OMD was differentially diagnosed based on the characteristic phenomenology of focal dystonia, such as stereotypy, task specificity, sensory tricks, overflow phenomenon, morning benefit, co-contraction, and EMG findings, as described in detail previously [8,9,11]. The main symptoms of the patients were masticatory disturbance (n = 146, 35.8%), discomfort and cosmetic problems associated with involuntary movement (n = 123, 30.1%), pain (n = 78, 19.1%), dysarthria (n = 68, 16.7%), and dysphagia (n = 41, 10.0%).

The inclusion criteria were as follows: (1) age over 18 years, (2) ability to be evaluated for OMDRS by interview or questionnaire, and (3) follow-up of 12 months or longer. The exclusion criteria were as follows: (1) generalized, functional [38], or significant dystonia-related neurological diseases in other body regions; (2) history of surgical procedures such as coronoidotomy [63,64] or deep brain stimulation; (3) good response to other therapies such as oral medicine, mouthpiece (sensory trick splint) [61], or muscle afferent block therapy [2,20]; (4) overseas resident, for whom regular follow-up and evaluation were not possible; and (5) common BoNT contraindications such as systemic neuromuscular junction disorders (myasthenia gravis, Lambert-Eaton syndrome, and amyotrophic lateral sclerosis), current or possible pregnancy, and lactation.

The patients were divided into six groups according to the six subtypes of OMD (jaw closing, tongue, jaw opening, jaw deviation, jaw protrusion, and lip dystonia) based on the direction of abnormal jaw movements (Table 1). If two or more subtypes coexisted in a patient, they were classified as having the most severe subtype [8,9,11].

Four hundred and eight patients with OMD were evaluated using the OMDRS (Figure S1) at baseline and endpoint or in stable condition. The endpoint was the time when the patient was satisfied with the therapeutic effect and BoNT therapy was completed. This means that the symptoms had subsided, and the BoNT injection was discontinued. Evaluation using the OMDRS was conducted one month after the last injection. In some patients, the symptoms had subsided and were being followed-up, but when the effect of BoNT wore off a little, they resumed injections. Patients in such stable condition on regular or additional BoNT injections were assessed by OMDRS one month after the last injection. Before the rating, the maximum occlusal force, maximum mouth opening, protrusion, and lateral movements, as well as protrusion or deviation of the tongue or lip were measured according to the subtype [9]. The maximum occlusal force was measured bilaterally on the molars three times using an occlusal force meter (GM10; Nagano Keiki Co., Tokyo, Japan) [9,39]. The patients were requested to speak or chew according to the video examination protocol, and the subsequent deviation was carefully rated. Regarding involuntary mouth closing (clenching), the patients were asked to close the mouth maximally and forcefully. Subsequently, the patients were asked the following question: "What is the percent force exerted when you close mouth involuntarily compared to the maximum bite force you have just tried?" [9].

The patients were interviewed to rate the severity, disability, and pain subscales. Questionnaires were then administered to the patients. The Japanese version of the OMDRS was used for 405 Japanese patients, whereas three international patients completed the English version of the OMDRS (Figure S1).

Improvement was calculated as the rate of decrease in the total OMDRS score. A partial responder was defined as a patient with less than 30% improvement.

Patients received an explanation of the treatment plan and provided written informed consent. This study was performed in accordance with the Declaration of Helsinki after approval from the institutional review board and ethics committee of Kyoto Medical Center (15-031).

5.2. BoNT Therapy

Before BoNT therapy was initiated, 3–5 mL of 0.5% lidocaine (Xylocaine; Sandoz K.K. Tokyo, Japan) was injected into the muscles with dystonia contracture to rule out patients whose symptoms were not caused by muscle tension [13,14,39]. Changes in involuntary movements and other symptoms were carefully examined after the lidocaine injection. If patients showed no changes in symptoms, other treatments were considered and no BoNT injections were performed. If patients showed improvement in symptoms under the effects of the local anesthetic, BoNT injections were administered [13,14].

BoNT injection methods have already been reported and discussed in detail for the lateral pterygoid [13,14,18,37], medial pterygoid [13,14,37], and tongue muscles [13,14,19]. BoNT (onabotulinumtoxinA; BOTOX®; Allergan, Irvine, CA, USA, AbbVie, North Chicago, IL, USA) was reconstituted with isotonic sodium chloride solution to reach a concentration of 2.5–5 units/0.1 mL. A disposable hypodermic needle electrode (TECA MyoJect Luer Lock, 37 mm × 25 G, 50 mm × 25 G; Natus Manufacturing Limited, Galway Gort, Ireland) was inserted into the target muscles. Correct placement of the needle electrode was confirmed under EMG guidance using an EMG instrument (Neuropack n1, MEM-8301, Nihon Kohden, Tokyo, Japan). After aspiration, BoNT was injected into the target muscles.

To prevent masticatory disturbance due to an excessively reduced bite force, the maximum occlusal force was measured on the bilateral molars using an occlusal force meter [13,14,39]. The muscles and doses of BoNT were individually determined for each patient based on their symptoms or occlusal force. The injections were continued until the patient was satisfied with the therapeutic effect and the injection was completed. The injection interval was 3–6 months depending on the patient's symptoms and requests.

5.3. Statistical Analysis

All statistical analyses were performed using the statistical software package, Statistical Package for the Social Sciences for Windows (version 24.0; SPSS Japan, Tokyo, Japan). The null hypothesis was rejected at the 5% significance level ($p < 0.05$). Differences among the six subtypes were statistically compared using one-way analysis of variance. The Bonferroni method was used as a post hoc test when analysis of variance revealed significant differences. Fisher's exact test and unpaired t-tests were used to assess the statistical significance of the differences in the distributions.

Supplementary Materials: The following supporting information can be downloaded at: https://www.mdpi.com/article/10.3390/toxins14100656/s1, Figure S1: Oromandibular Dystonia Rating Scale (OMDRS).

Funding: This research was funded by JSPS KAKENHI (grant numbers JP24592946 and JP22111201).

Institutional Review Board Statement: This study was conducted in accordance with the guidelines of the Declaration of Helsinki and approved by the Institutional Review Board and Ethics Committee of Kyoto Medical Center (15-031).

Informed Consent Statement: The patients received an explanation of the treatment plan and provided written informed consent.

Data Availability Statement: The raw data supporting the conclusions of this article will be made available by the authors, without undue reservation, to any qualified researcher.

Conflicts of Interest: The author declares no conflict of interest. The sponsor had no role in the design, execution, interpretation, or writing of the study.

References

1. Albanese, A.; Bhatia, K.; Bressman, S.B.; Delong, M.R.; Fahn, S.; Fung, V.S.; Hallett, M.; Jankovic, J.; Jinnah, H.A.; Klein, C.; et al. Phenomenology and classification of dystonia: A consensus up date. *Mov. Disord.* **2013**, *28*, 863–873. [CrossRef] [PubMed]
2. Yoshida, K.; Kaji, R.; Kubori, T.; Kohara, N.; Iizuka, T.; Kimura, J. Muscle afferent block for the treatment of oromandibular dystonia. *Mov. Disord.* **1998**, *13*, 699–705. [CrossRef] [PubMed]
3. Bakke, M.; Larsen, B.M.; Dalager, T.; Møller, E. Oromandibular dystonia–functional and clinical characteristics: A report on 21 cases. *Oral Surg. Oral Med. Oral Pathol. Oral Radiol.* **2013**, *115*, e21–e26. [CrossRef] [PubMed]
4. Sinclair, C.F.; Gurey, L.E.; Blitzer, A. Oromandibular dystonia: Long-term management with botulinum toxin. *Laryngoscope* **2013**, *123*, 3078–3083. [CrossRef] [PubMed]
5. Skármeta, N.P.; Espinoza-Mellado, P.; Chana, P. Orofacial dystonia and other oromandibular movement disorders. In *Dystonia*; Rizk, T.M.G., Ed.; IntechOpen: London, UK, 2018. [CrossRef]
6. Comella, C.L. Systematic review of botulinum toxin treatment for oromandibular dystonia. *Toxicon* **2018**, *147*, 96–99. [CrossRef] [PubMed]
7. Dadgardoust, P.D.; Rosales, R.L.; Asuncion, R.M.; Dressler, D. Botulinum neurotoxin a therapy efficacy and safety for oromandibular dystonia: A meta-analysis. *J. Neural Transm.* **2019**, *126*, 141–148. [CrossRef] [PubMed]
8. Yoshida, K. Oromandibular dystonia screening questionnaire for differential diagnosis. *Clin. Oral Investig.* **2019**, *23*, 405–411. [CrossRef]
9. Yoshida, K. Development and validation of a disease-specific oromandibular dystonia rating scale (OMDRS). *Front. Neurol.* **2020**, *11*, 583177. [CrossRef]
10. Scorr, L.M.; Factor, S.A.; Parra, S.P.; Kaye, R.; Paniello, R.C.; Norris, S.A.; Perlmutter, J.S.; Bäumer, T.; Usnich, T.; Berman, B.D.; et al. Oromandibular dystonia: A clinical examination of 2020 cases. *Front. Neurol.* **2021**, *12*, 700714. [CrossRef]
11. Yoshida, K. Prevalence and incidence of oromandibular dystonia: An oral and maxillofacial surgery service-based study. *Clin. Oral Investig.* **2021**, *25*, 5755–5764. [CrossRef]
12. Yoshida, K. Behandlungsstrategien bei oromandibulärer Dystonie. *Fortschr. Neurol. Psychiatr.* **2021**, *89*, 1562–1572. [CrossRef] [PubMed]
13. Yoshida, K. Botulinum toxin therapy for oromandibular dystonia and other movement disorders in the stomatognathic system. *Toxins* **2022**, *14*, 282. [CrossRef] [PubMed]
14. Yoshida, K.; Botulinum Toxin Therapy for Oromandibular Dystonia. Scholarly Community Encyclopedia. 2022. Available online: https://encyclopedia.pub/entry/23511 (accessed on 1 August 2022).
15. Nutt, J.G.; Muenter, M.D.; Aronson, A.; Kurland, L.T.; Melton, L.J., 3rd. Epidemiology of focal and generalized dystonia in Rochester, Minnesota. *Mov. Disord.* **1988**, *3*, 188–194. [CrossRef] [PubMed]
16. Steeves, T.D.; Day, L.; Dykeman, J.; Jette, N.; Pringsheim, T. The prevalence of primary dystonia: A systematic review and meta-analysis. *Mov. Disord.* **2012**, *27*, 1789–1796. [CrossRef] [PubMed]
17. Yoshida, K.; Iizuka, T. Botulinum toxin treatment for upper airway collapse resulting from temporomandibular joint dislocation due to jaw-opening dystonia. *Cranio* **2006**, *24*, 217–222. [CrossRef] [PubMed]
18. Yoshida, K. Botulinum neurotoxin injection for the treatment of recurrent temporomandibular joint dislocation with and without neurogenic muscular hyperactivity. *Toxins* **2018**, *10*, 174. [CrossRef]
19. Yoshida, K. Botulinum neurotoxin therapy for lingual dystonia using an individualized injection method based on clinical features. *Toxins* **2019**, *11*, 51. [CrossRef] [PubMed]
20. Yoshida, K.; Kaji, R.; Shibasaki, H.; Iizuka, T. Factors influencing the therapeutic effect of muscle afferent block for oromandibular dystonia and dyskinesia: Implications for their distinct pathophysiology. *Int. J. Oral Maxillofac. Surg.* **2002**, *31*, 499–505. [CrossRef]
21. Merz, R.I.; Deakin, J.; Hawthorne, M.R. Oromandibular dystonia questionnaire (OMDQ-25): A valid and reliable instrument for measuring health-related quality of life. *Clin. Otolaryngol.* **2010**, *35*, 390–396. [CrossRef]
22. Albanese, A.; Sorbo, F.D.; Comella, C.; Jinnah, H.A.; Mink, J.W.; Post, B.; Vidailhet, M.; Volkmann, J.; Warner, T.T.; Leentjens, A.F.G.; et al. Dystonia rating scales: Critique and recommendations. *Mov. Disord.* **2013**, *28*, 874–883. [CrossRef]
23. Del Sorbo, F.; Albanese, A. Botulinum neurotoxins for the treatment of focal dystonias: Review of rating tools used in clinical trials. *Toxicon* **2015**, *107*, 89–97. [CrossRef]
24. Bhattacharyya, N.; Tarsy, D. Impact on quality of life of botulinum toxin treatments for spasmodic dysphonia and oromandibular dystonia. *Arch. Otolaryngol. Head Neck Surg.* **2001**, *127*, 389–392. [CrossRef] [PubMed]
25. Charous, S.J.; Comella, C.L.; Fan, W. Jaw-opening dystonia: Quality of life after botulinum toxin injections. *Ear Nose Throat J.* **2011**, *90*, E9–E12. [CrossRef] [PubMed]

26. Page, A.D.; Siegel, L.; Jog, M. Self-Rated communication-related quality of life of individuals with oromandibular dystonia receiving botulinum toxin injections. *Am. J. Speech Lang. Pathol.* **2017**, *26*, 674–681. [CrossRef]
27. Page, A.D.; Elhayek, N.; Baylor, C.; Adams, S.; Jog, M.; Yorkston, K. Exploring the psychosocial impact of botulinum toxin type A injections for individuals with oromandibular dystonia: A qualitative study of patients' experiences. *Am. J. Speech Lang. Pathol.* **2021**, *30*, 1314–1328. [CrossRef]
28. Kuyper, D.J.; Parra, V.; Aerts, S.; Okun, M.S.; Kluger, B.M. The non-motor manifestations of dystonia: A systematic review. *Mov. Disord.* **2011**, *26*, 1206–1217. [CrossRef] [PubMed]
29. Klingelhoefer, L.; Kaiser, M.; Sauerbier, A.; Untucht, R.; Wienecke, M.; Mammadova, K.; Falkenburger, B.; Gregor, O.; Chaudhuri, K.R.; Reichmann, H. Emotional well-being and pain could be a greater determinant of quality of life compared to motor severity in cervical dystonia. *J. Neural. Transm.* **2021**, *128*, 305–314. [CrossRef]
30. Ndukwe, I.; O'Riordan, S.; Walsh, C.B.; Hutchinson, M. Trust the patient not the doctor: The determinants of quality of life in cervical dystonia. *Front. Neurol.* **2020**, *11*, 991. [CrossRef]
31. Junker, J.; Berman, B.D.; Hall, J.; Wahba, D.W.; Brandt, V.; Perlmutter, J.S.; Jankovic, J.; Malaty, I.A.; Shukla, A.W.; Reich, S.G.; et al. Quality of life in isolated dystonia: Non-motor manifestations matter. *J. Neurol. Neurosurg. Psychiatry* **2021**, *92*, 622–628. [CrossRef]
32. Costanzo, M.; Belvisi, D.; Berardelli, I.; Maraone, A.; Baione, V.; Ferrazzano, G.; Cutrona, C.; Leodori, G.; Pasquini, M.; Conte, A.; et al. Effect of botulinum toxin on non-motor symptoms in cervical dystonia. *Toxins* **2021**, *13*, 647. [CrossRef]
33. Nastasi, L.; Mostile, G.; Nicoletti, A.; Zappia, M.; Reggio, E.; Catania, S. Effect of botulinum toxin treatment on quality of life in patients with isolated lingual dystonia and oromandibular dystonia affecting the tongue. *J. Neurol.* **2016**, *263*, 1702–1708. [CrossRef]
34. Scorr, L.M.; Silver, M.R.; Hanfelt, J.; Sperin, E.; Freeman, A.; Jinnah, H.A.; Factor, S.A. Pilot single-blind trial of AbobotulinumtoxinA in oromandibular dystonia. *Neurotherapeutics* **2018**, *15*, 452–458. [CrossRef] [PubMed]
35. Cronbach, L.J. Coefficient alpha and the internal structure of tests. *Psychometrica* **1951**, *16*, 297–334. [CrossRef]
36. Cano, S.J.; Warner, T.T.; Linacre, J.M.; Bhatia, K.P.; Thompson, A.J.; Fitzpatrick, R.; Hobart, J.C. Capturing the true burden of dystonia on patients: The Cervical Dystonia Impact Profile (CDIP-58). *Neurology* **2004**, *63*, 1629–1633. [CrossRef] [PubMed]
37. Yoshida, K. How do I inject botulinum toxin into the lateral and medial pterygoid muscles? *Mov. Disord. Clin. Pract.* **2016**, *4*, 285. [CrossRef] [PubMed]
38. Yoshida, K. Clinical characteristics of functional movement disorders in the stomatognathic system. *Front. Neurol.* **2020**, *11*, 23. [CrossRef]
39. Yoshida, K. Effects of botulinum toxin type A on pain among trigeminal neuralgia, myofascial temporomandibular disorders, and oromandibular dystonia. *Toxins* **2021**, *13*, 605. [CrossRef]
40. Berardelli, I.; Ferrazzano, G.; Pasquini, M.; Biondi, M.; Berardelli, A.; Fabbrini, G. Clinical course of psychiatric disorders in patients with cervical dystonia. *Psychiatry Res.* **2015**, *229*, 583–585. [CrossRef] [PubMed]
41. Hallett, M. Neurophysiology of dystonia: The role of inhibition. *Neurobiol. Dis.* **2011**, *42*, 177–184. [CrossRef]
42. Stamelou, M.; Edwards, M.J.; Hallett, M.; Bhatia, K.P. The non-motor syndrome of primary dystonia: Clinical and pathophysio logical implications. *Brain* **2012**, *135*, 1668–1681. [CrossRef]
43. Fabbrini, G.; Berardelli, I.; Moretti, G.; Pasquini, M.; Bloise, M.; Colosimo, C.; Biondi, M.; Berardelli, A. Psychiatric disorders in adult-onset focal dystonia: A case-control study. *Mov. Disord.* **2010**, *25*, 459–465. [CrossRef]
44. Singer, C.; Papapetropoulos, S. A comparison of jaw-closing and jaw-opening idiopathic oromandibular dystonia. *Parkinsonism Relat. Disord.* **2006**, *12*, 115–118. [CrossRef] [PubMed]
45. Yoshida, K. Computer-aided design/computer-assisted manufacture-derived needle guide for injection of botulinum toxin into the lateral pterygoid muscle in patients with oromandibular dystonia. *J. Oral Facial Pain Headache* **2018**, *32*, e13–e21. [CrossRef]
46. Yoshida, K. An electromyographic study on the superior head of the lateral pterygoid muscle during mastication from the standpoint of condylar movement. *J. Jpn. Prosthodont. Soc.* **1992**, *36*, 110–120.
47. Yoshida, K. Eigenschaften der Kaumuskelaktivität während verschiedener Unterkieferbewegungen bei Patienten mit Diskusverlagerung ohne Reposition. *Stomatologie* **1999**, *96*, 107–121.
48. Yoshida, K. Masticatory muscle responses associated with unloading of biting force during food crushing. *J. Oral Rehabil.* **1998**, *25*, 830–837. [CrossRef] [PubMed]
49. Usui, A.; Akita, K.; Yamaguchi, K. An anatomic study of the divisions of the lateral pterygoid muscle based on the findings of the origins and insertions. *Surg. Radiol. Anat.* **2008**, *30*, 327–333. [CrossRef] [PubMed]
50. Stöckle, M.; Fanghänel, J.; Knüttel, H.; Alamanos, C.; Behr, M. The morphological variations of the lateral pterygoid muscle: A systematic review. *Ann. Anat.* **2019**, *222*, 79–87. [CrossRef]
51. Yoshida, K. Multilingual website and cyberconsultations for oromandibular dystonia. *Neurol. Int.* **2018**, *10*, 7536. [CrossRef]
52. Logroscino, G.; Livrea, P.; Anaclerio, D.; Aniello, M.S.; Benedetto, G.; Cazzato, G.; Giampietro, L.; Manobianca, G.; Marra, M.; Martino, D.; et al. Agreement among neurologista on the clinical diagnosis of dystonia at different body sites. *J. Neurol. Neurosurg. Psychiatry* **2003**, *74*, 348–350. [CrossRef]
53. Saraf, U.; Chandarana, M.; Divya, K.P.; Krishnan, S. Oromandibular dystonia—A systematic review. *Ann. Indian Acad. Neurol.* **2022**, *25*, 26–34. [CrossRef] [PubMed]
54. Yoshida, K. Involuntary Movements of the Stomatognathic Region. Available online: https://sites.google.com/site/oromandibulardystoniaenglish (accessed on 1 August 2022).

55. Jankovic, J.; Orman, J. Botulinum a toxin for cranial-cervical dystonia: A double-blind, placebo-controlled study. *Neurology* **1987**, *37*, 616–623. [CrossRef] [PubMed]
56. Blitzer, A.; Brin, M.; Greene, P.E.; Fahn, S. Botulinum toxin injection for the treatment of oromandibular dystonia. *Ann. Otol. Rhinol. Laryngol.* **1989**, *98*, 93–97. [CrossRef] [PubMed]
57. Hermanowicz, N.; Truong, D.D. Treatment of oromandibular dystonia with botulinum toxin. *Laryngoscope* **1991**, *101*, 1216–1218. [CrossRef] [PubMed]
58. Tan, E.K.; Jankovic, J. Botulinum toxin A in patients with oromandibular dystonia: Long-term follow-up. *Neurology* **1999**, *53*, 2102–2107. [CrossRef]
59. Rosales, R.L.; Ng, A.R.; Santos, M.M.D.-D.; Fernandez, H.H. The broadening application of chemodenervation in X-linked dystonia-parkinsonism (Part II): An open-label experience with botulinum toxin-A (Dysport®) injections for oromandibular, lingual, and truncal-axial dystonias. *Int. J. Neurosci.* **2011**, *121* (Suppl. S1), 44–56. [CrossRef]
60. Yoshida, K.; Kaji, R.; Takagi, A.; Iizuka, T. Customized EMG needle insertion guide for the muscle afferent block of jaw-deviation and jaw-opening dystonias. *Oral Surg. Oral Med. Oral Pathol. Oral Radiol. Endod.* **1999**, *88*, 664–669. [CrossRef]
61. Yoshida, K. Sensory trick splint as a multimodal therapy for oromandibular dystonia. *J. Prosthodont. Res.* **2018**, *62*, 239–244. [CrossRef] [PubMed]
62. De Meyer, M.; Vereecke, L.; Bottenberg, P.; Jacquet, W.; Sims, A.B.; Santens, P. Oral appliances in the treatment of oromandibular dystonia: A systematic review. *Acta Neurol. Belg.* **2020**, *120*, 831–836. [CrossRef] [PubMed]
63. Yoshida, K. Coronoidotomy as treatment for trismus due to jaw-closing oromandibular dystonia. *Mov. Disord.* **2006**, *21*, 1028–1031. [CrossRef]
64. Yoshida, K. Surgical intervention for oromandibular dystonia-related limited mouth opening: Long-term follow-up. *J. Cranio-Maxillofac. Surg.* **2017**, *45*, 56–62. [CrossRef] [PubMed]
65. Yoshida, K. Mouth opening retaining appliance after coronoidotomy for the treatment of trismus: Effects on pain during postoperative training and maximal extent of mouth opening. *Clin. Surg.* **2020**, *5*, 2737. [CrossRef]
66. Ondo, W.G.; Simmons, J.H.; Shahid, M.H.; Hashem, V.; Hunter, C.; Jankovic, J. Onabotulinum toxin-A injections for sleep bruxism: A double-blind, placebo-controlled study. *Neurology* **2018**, *90*, e559–e564. [CrossRef] [PubMed]
67. De la Torre Canales, G.; Poluha, R.L.; Pinzón, N.A.; DaSilva, B.R.; Almeida, A.M.; Ernberg, M.; Manso, A.C.; Bonjardim, L.R.; Rizzatti-Barbosa, C.M. Efficacy of botulinum toxin type-A I in the improvement of mandibular motion and muscle sensibility in myofascial pain TMD Subjects: A randomized controlled trial. *Toxins* **2022**, *14*, 441. [CrossRef] [PubMed]
68. Ferrillo, M.; Ammendolia, A.; Paduano, S.; Calafiore, D.; Marotta, N.; Migliario, M.; Fortunato, L.; Giudice, A.; Michelotti, A.; de Sire, A. Efficacy of rehabilitation on reducing pain in muscle-related temporomandibular disorders: A systematic review and meta-analysis of randomized controlled trials. *J. Back Musculoskelet. Rehabil.* **2022**, *35*, 921–936. [CrossRef] [PubMed]

toxins MDPI

Article

Effect of Botulinum Toxin Injection on EMG Activity and Bite Force in Masticatory Muscle Disorder: A Randomized Clinical Trial

Victoria Sitnikova [1], Antti Kämppi [1,*], Olli Teronen [2] and Pentti Kemppainen [1,3]

1 Department of Oral and Maxillofacial Diseases, Faculty of Medicine, University of Helsinki, 00280 Helsinki, Finland
2 Dental Clinic, Private Practice Mehiläinen, 00100 Helsinki, Finland
3 Oral and Dental Centre, Helsinki University Central Hospital (HUCH), 00290 Helsinki, Finland
* Correspondence: antti.kamppi@helsinki.fi; Tel.: +358-2941911

Abstract: Botulinum toxin type A (BoNT-A) is increasingly used in treating masticatory muscle pain disorder; however, safe doses and reinjection intervals still need to be established. The purpose of this randomized clinical trial was to evaluate the degree and duration of the impairment of masticatory muscle performance. Fifty-seven subjects were randomly divided into two groups: one of which received BoNT-A first ($n = 28$) while the other received saline first ($n = 29$), with the cross-over being in week 16, and a total follow-up period of 32 weeks. A total dose of 50 U of BoNT-A was injected in the masseter and temporal muscles bilaterally. Electromyographic (EMG) activity and bite forces were assessed. A significant reduction in EMG activity was observed up to week 18 ($p \leq 001$), with total recovery at week 33. A significant reduction in maximum bite force was observed up to week 11 ($p \leq 005$), with total recovery at week 25. In conclusion, when treating masticatory muscle pain disorder with 50 U of BoNT-A, a reinjection interval of 33 weeks can be considered safe since the recovery of muscle function occurs by that time.

Keywords: temporomandibular disorders; masticatory muscle disorder; myofascial pain; chronic pain; botulinum toxin type A

Key Contribution: Masticatory muscle performance diminishes significantly after the injections of 50 U of botulinum toxin type A. The recovery occurs in 33 weeks.

Citation: Sitnikova, V.; Kämppi, A.; Teronen, O.; Kemppainen, P. Effect of Botulinum Toxin Injection on EMG Activity and Bite Force in Masticatory Muscle Disorder: A Randomized Clinical Trial. *Toxins* **2022**, *14*, 545. https://doi.org/10.3390/toxins14080545

Received: 1 July 2022
Accepted: 8 August 2022
Published: 10 August 2022

1. Introduction

Masticatory muscle disorder is a common pain condition classified as temporomandibular disorder (TMD) [1]. It can be subclassified into myalgia, myofascial pain, and headache attributed to TMD. Noninvasive therapies, including behavior therapy, pharmacotherapy, physical therapy, and occlusal appliances are effective in most cases. Still, approximately 10% of TMD patients develop a disorder associated with chronic orofacial pain [2,3]. For these patients, injections of botulinum toxin A (BoNT-A) have been suggested as a treatment of choice given its relaxing and analgesic effect. The use of BoNT-A has significantly increased over recent years. However, its safety when injected systematically remains unclear.

Most of the studies concerning botulinum toxin for treating TMD concentrate on the drug's effect on pain findings [4–6]. Some temporary and mostly insignificant adverse effects had been reported by the patients according to several studies, such as pain at the injection site, bruising, muscle weakness, and undesirable muscle paralysis [7,8]. In virtually all studies, they are reported as qualitative results, limited to self-reporting, concern the single injection of the current study, and are caused by the puncture itself. However, the objective evaluation of the drug's effect on muscle and surrounding structures should also be taken into consideration since it is a toxin that causes muscle paralysis and the accumulation of physiological changes due to systematic injections might lead to unfavorable long-term side effects harming the masticatory system.

It is generally thought that muscle function is restored in 3 to 6 months after the injections [9,10]. However, in studies where muscle functional effect was evaluated using electromyography (EMG), the effect of the drug was present for up to 12 months [11]. The studies evaluating bony changes corroborate the drug's long-lasting hidden effect [12,13]. Permanent damage to neuromuscular function has also been considered [14]. The effect is likely to be cumulative if the structures are not allowed to recover before the repeated injections [15]. Thus, understanding the muscle recovery rate is important to establish safe intervals for reinjections.

In this randomized controlled trial, the recovery of muscle function after a single injection of 50 U of BoNT-A was quantitively evaluated. The parameters used in this research are EMG and bite force.

2. Results

2.1. Patients

The process from patient recruitment to analysis is illustrated as a flow diagram (Figure 1). Twenty-eight participants included in the analysis received BoNT-A first (the BS group) and twenty-nine received saline first (the SB group). The demographic and diagnostic characteristics of the subjects appear in Tables 1 and 2. Most patients were female, (82.5%) with a mean age of 38.2 (range 22 to 64 years). Educational level was high, with 26.3% having graduated from the university of applied science and 38.6% from the university. The majority were employed.

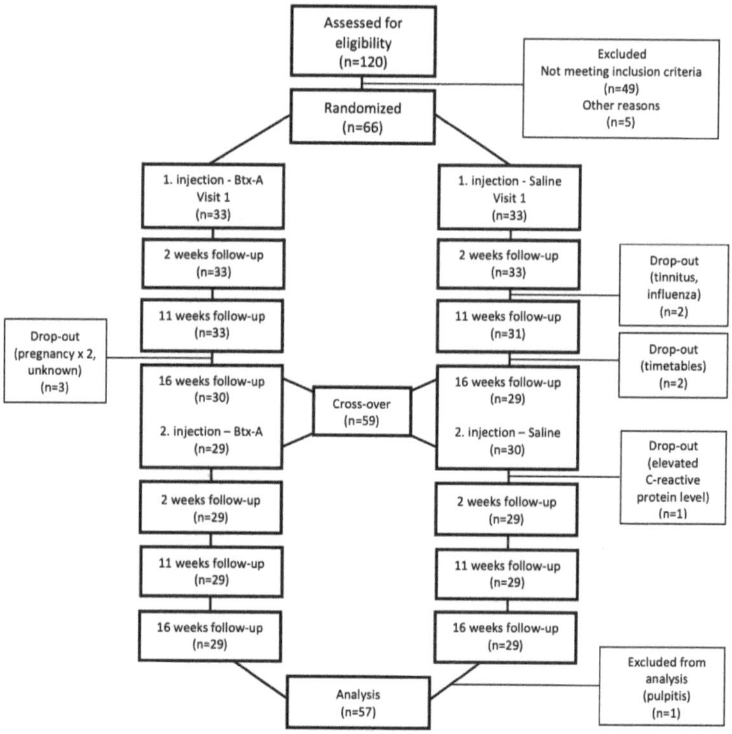

Figure 1. CONSORT diagram for participant enrollment.

Table 1. Patient sociodemographic characteristics.

Sociodemographic Characteristics	% (n)
Gender	
Male (age 33.8 ± 8.5 [22–51])	17.5 (10)
Female (age 39.2 ± 10.5 [24–64])	82.5 (47)
All (age 38.2 ± 10.4 [22–64])	100.0 (57)
Education	
High school	5.3 (3)
Vocational school	24.6 (14)
Polytechnic	26.3 (15)
University	38.6 (22)
Not reported	5.3 (3)
Occupation	
Student	15.8 (9)
Employed (Entrepreneur)	75.4 (43)
Working at home	3.5 (2)
Not reported	5.3 (3)
Marital status	
Married	35.1 (20)
Cohabiting	24.6 (14)
Divorced	15.8 (9)
Never married	19.3 (11)
Not reported	5.3 (3)

Table 2. Patient diagnostic characteristics.

Diagnostic Characteristics	% (n)
DC/TMD diagnosis	
Myalgia	46.4(52)
Myofascial pain with referral	18.8 (21)
Headache attributed to TMD	21.4 (24)
Arthralgia right	2.7 (3)
Arthralgia left	7.1 (8)
Other *	3.6 (4)
Pain chronicity	
1 to <5 years	24.6 (14)
5 to <10 years	24.6 (14)
≥10 years	47.4 (27)
Not reported	3.5 (2)
Pain frequency	
Persistent	40.4 (23)
Recurrent	54.4 (31)
One-time	1.8 (1)
Not reported	3.5 (2)

* According to the History questionnaire of the Research Diagnostic Criteria for Temporomandibular Disorders patients have had pain in the face, jaw, temple, in front of the ear, or the ear in the past month. No TMD diagnosis was obtained based on clinical examination.

Fifty-two patients (91.2%) were diagnosed with TMD-related myalgia, of which, twenty-one (38.2% of all patients) were diagnosed with myofascial pain with a referral. Twenty-four patients (42.1%) had headaches attributed to TMD. Three patients were diagnosed with right arthralgia and eight with left arthralgia. Almost half of the patients (47.4%) had suffered from pain symptoms for at least ten years. Twenty-three patients (40.4%) reported persistent pain symptoms and thirty-one (54.4%) reported recurrent pain symptoms.

2.2. Electromyography (EMG)

The greatest decrease in EMG activity was observed two weeks after the BoNT-A injections (Figure 2). The effect of the drug attenuated continuously up to week 32.

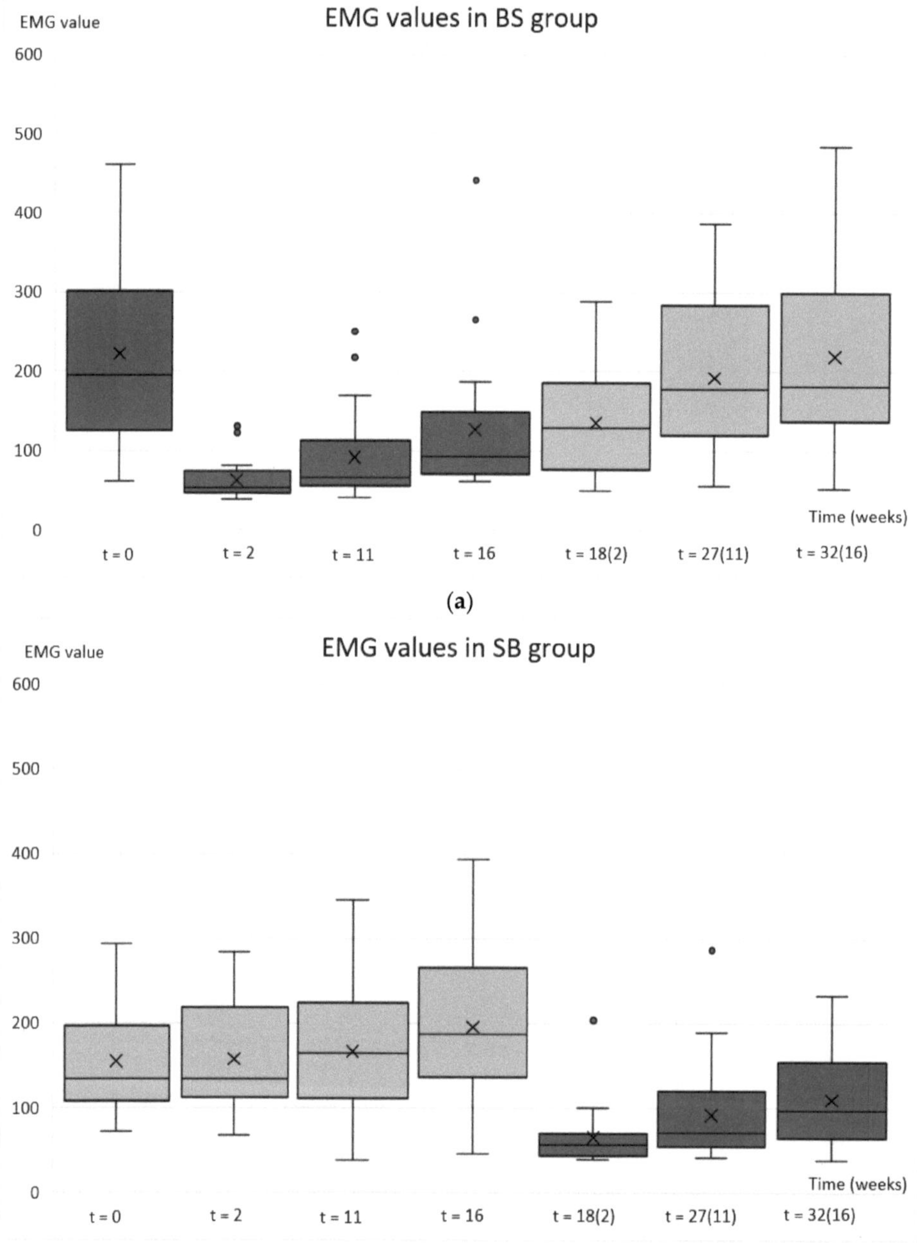

(b)

Figure 2. Box plots of the average electromyography (EMG) values of the masseter muscle after botulinum toxin and saline injections. The BS group (**a**) botulinum toxin injected at the baseline and saline at the 16-week follow-up; the SB group (**b**) saline injected at the baseline and botulinum toxin at the 16-week follow-up. The week calculated from the second injection is marked in brackets. For each box plot, maximum and minimum, 25th and 75th percentiles, median (solid line inside the box), mean (cross inside the box), and outliers (dots) are presented.

The mean EMGmax values over time for the BS group were 222 mV (day 0), 62 mV (week 2), 92 mV (week 11), 126 mV (week 16), 135 mV (week 18, i.e., 2 weeks after the second injection), 191 mV (week 27, i.e., 11 weeks after the second injection), and 219 mV (week 32, i.e., 16 weeks after the second injection) (Figure 2a). The mean EMGmax values over time for the SB group were 155 mV (day 0), 158 mV (week 2), 170 mV (week 11), 195 mV (week 16), 65 mV (week 18, i.e., 2 weeks after the second injection), 93 mV (week 27, i.e., 11 weeks after the second injection), and 112 mV (week 32, i.e., 16 weeks after the second injection) (Figure 2b).

Comparing EMGmax values within the BS group between time-points showed a highly significant decrease ($p \leq 0.001$) in EMGmax values on follow-up weeks 2, 11, 16, and 18 compared to the values before the BoNT-A injection (Table 3). EMGmax values were decreased by 72% at the 2-week follow-up, 59% at the 11-week follow-up, 43% at the 16-week follow-up, 39% at the 18-week follow-up, 14% at the 27-week follow-up, and 1% at the 32-week follow-up. The linearity was observed in the recovery of EMGmax values and full recovery was expected by week 33 based on the forecast function (Figure 3a).

Table 3. Comparison of EMGmax and maximum bite force values within one group between time-points. BS group: botulinum toxin injected at the baseline and saline at the 16-week follow-up; SB group: saline injected at the baseline and botulinum toxin at the 16-week follow-up. The week calculated from the second injection is marked in brackets.

	p Values *					
	Time Range (Weeks)					
	0–2	0–11	0–16	0–18 (2)	0–27 (11)	0–32 (16)
EMG BS group	0.000	0.000	0.000	0.001	0.122	0.994
EMG SB group	0.582	0.079	0.005	<0.001	<0.001	<0.001
FORCE BS group	<0.001	0.002	0.167	0.109	0.838	0.885
FORCE SB group	0.084	0.922	0.945	<0.001	0.025	0.520

* Wilcoxon Sign Rank exact test.

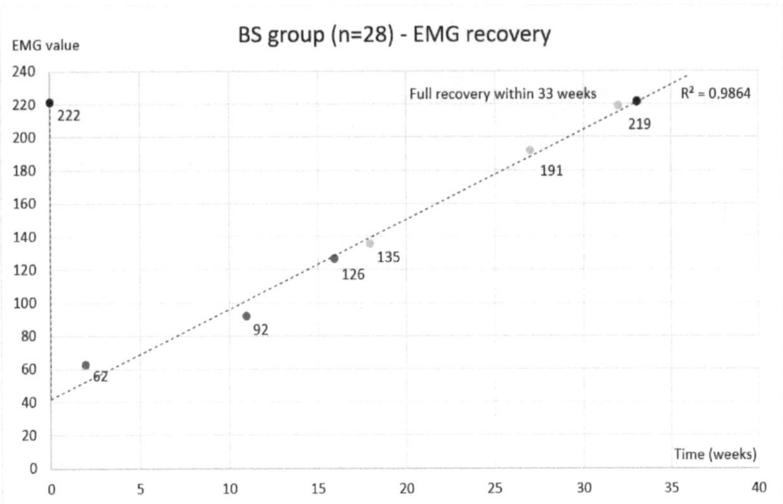

(a)

Figure 3. *Cont.*

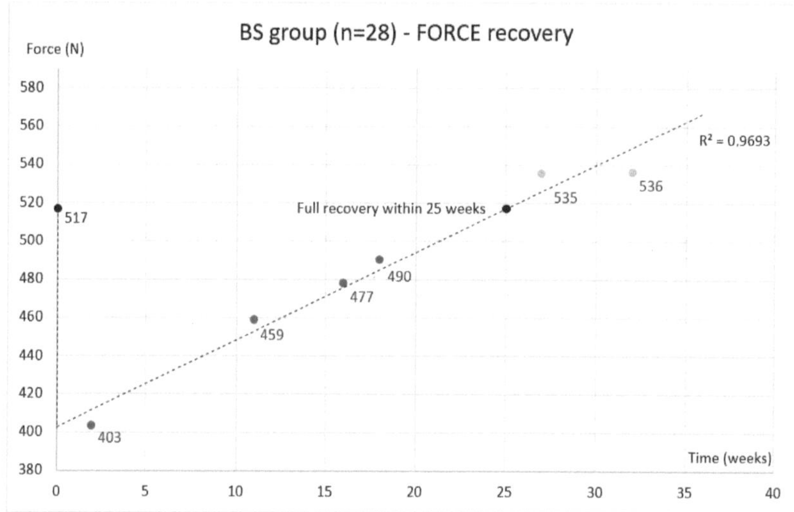

(**b**)

Figure 3. Regression lines for EMG (**a**) and bite force (**b**) mean values after botulinum toxin injection. BS group: botulinum toxin injected at the baseline and saline at the 16-week follow-up.

Comparing the EMGmax values within the SB group between time-points showed an increase in EMGmax after saline injection (Figure 2b). The difference was highly significant at the 16-week follow-up compared to the baseline ($p_{0-16} = 0.005$) (Table 3). The increase in EMGmax values was also noticeable at the 11-week follow-up, even though statistically non-significant ($p_{0-11} = 0.079$). A highly significant decrease ($p \leq 0.001$) in EMGmax values was observed after the second injection in follow-up weeks 18, 27, and 32 (i.e., 2, 11, and 16 after the BoNT-A injection). This is consistent with the findings of the BS group.

There were no great differences in EMGrest values over time either in the BS or SB groups; the values ranged from 38 mV to 41 mV.

2.3. *Bite Force*

Regarding bite force, the average decrease of 114 N was achieved with 50 U of BoNT-A. As with the EMG, the lowest value was obtained two weeks after the drug injection. The effect of the drug attenuates continuously up to week 27 (Figure 4).

The mean maximum bite force values over time for the BS group were 517 N (day 0), 403 N (week 2), 459 N (week 11), 477 N (week 16), 490 N (week 18, i.e., 2 weeks after the second injection), 535 N (27 weeks, i.e., 11 weeks after the second injection), and 536 N (32 weeks, i.e., 16 weeks after the second injection) (Figure 4a). The mean maximum bite force values over time for the SB group were 497 N (day 0), 508 N (week 2), 478 N (week 11), 486 N (week 16), 399 N (week 18, i.e., 2 weeks after the second injection), 427 N (27 weeks, i.e., 11 weeks after the second injection), and 453 N (32 weeks, i.e., 16 weeks after the second injection) (Figure 4b).

Comparing the maximum bite force values within the BS group between time-points showed a significant decrease at the 2 ($p_{0-2} \leq 0.001$) and 11 week ($p_{0-11} = 0.002$) follow-up compared to baseline (Table 3). Bite force values were decreased by 22% at the 2-week follow-up, 11% at the 11-week follow-up, 8% at the 16-week follow-up, and 5% at the 18-week follow-up. Compared to the baseline, 3% higher values at the 27-week follow-up and 4% at the 32-week follow-up were observed (Figure 4a). As with EMGmax values, the linearity was observed in the recovery of bite force and full recovery occurred at 25 weeks after BoNT-A injections based on the forecast function (Figure 3b).

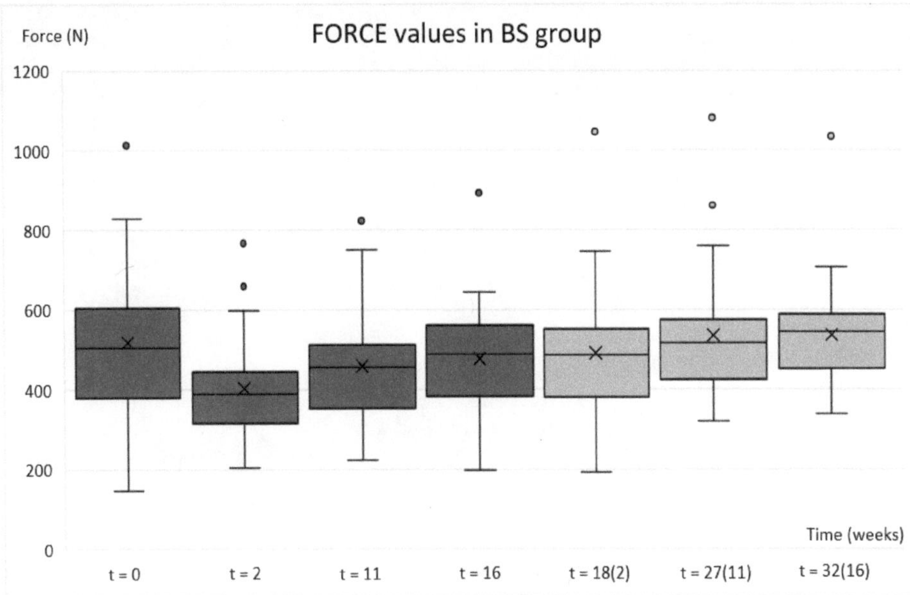

(a)

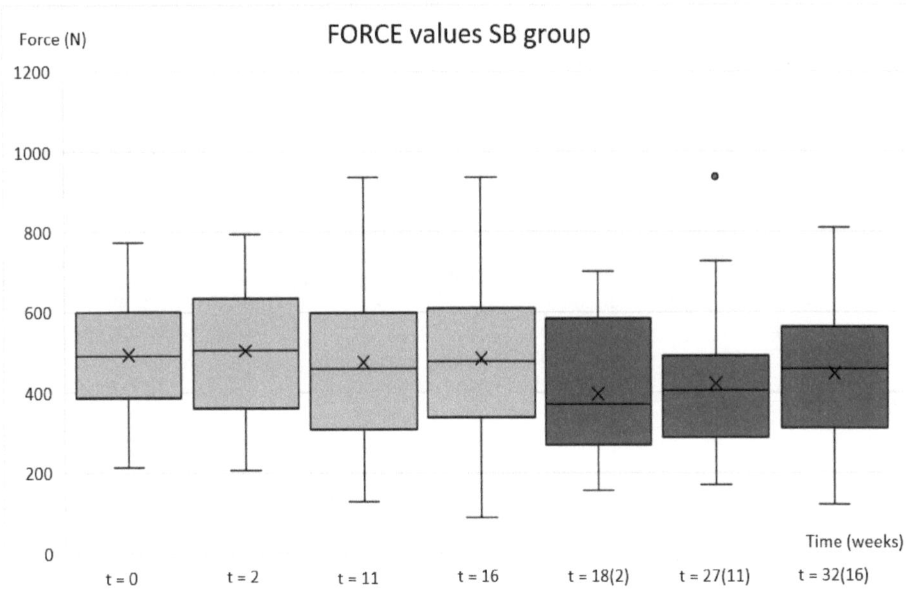

(b)

Figure 4. Box plots of bite force values after botulinum toxin and saline injections. BS group (**a**) botulinum toxin injected at the baseline and saline at the 16-week follow-up; SB group (**b**) saline injected at the baseline and botulinum toxin at the 16-week follow-up. The week calculated from the second injection is marked in brackets. For each box plot, maximum and minimum, 25th and 75th percentiles, median (solid line inside the box), mean (cross inside the box), and outliers (dots) are presented.

When maximum bite force values were compared within the SB group, no significant changes in values were observed after the saline injection. However, a significant decrease in bite force was noticed 2 weeks and 11 weeks after the BoNT-A injections ($p_{0\text{–}18} \leq 0.001$ and $p_{0\text{–}27} = 0.025$) (Table 3).

2.4. Harm

A total of 3 patients out of 59 reported harm after the BoNT-A injections. One patient reported smile asymmetry ten days after the injections, indicating that mimic muscles might have been involved. The recovery occurred within eight weeks. One patient reported the onset of migraine a few days after the BoNT-A injections and another reported tinnitus and pain symptoms in both ears, with the symptoms being gone at two weeks' follow-up.

3. Discussion

BoNT-A has gained a lot of interest in treating masticatory muscle pain conditions. Along with its analgesic effect, BoNT-A also causes structural and functional changes in muscle tissue, which are considered adverse reactions [7]. There are only a few studies evaluating the recovery of muscle along with pain symptoms [16–18]. EMG and bite force are both important parameters in evaluating masticatory muscle performance and the measurement methods are reliable, convenient, and safe. In addition, decreased EMG implies that neuromuscular junctions have not been restored, which directly reflects BoNT-A's denervation effect [14]. Our study showed that the recovery of EMG occurs by 33 weeks and bite-force by 25 weeks after a moderate dose of BoNT-A.

The present study supports previous findings concerning the significant decrease in EMG values after BoNT-A injections. However, the recovery course and time differ slightly. In our study, the maximum decrease of 72% of EMG of the masseter muscle was observed two weeks after the injection of 16.7 U into the masseter muscle and a significant reduction was still present 18 weeks later. The effect of BoNT-A was also noticeable 27 weeks after the injections with a total recovery taking 33 weeks. De la Torre Canales et al. reported about an 80% decrease in EMG values 28 days after the injections of 30 U of BoNT-A, with a total recovery after 180 days [16]. Compared to our study, the recovery of EMG was achieved earlier with a bigger dose. Kurtoglu et al. reported significantly lower EMG activity on day 14, but not on day 28 after the injection of 30 U of BoNT-A [18]. Such a rapid recovery is somewhat at odds with our findings.

Interestingly, EMGmax values increased slightly after saline injections in the SB group. In this blinded research setting, the subject might test the effect of the treatment by testing their muscle function, which might further increase the tonus of the jaw-closing muscles. This effect of the intervention itself is clinically not significant. However, this finding might indicate that EMG values would still be decreased 33 weeks after the drug injection when the effect of the intervention itself is eliminated.

Regarding maximum bite force, a 22% reduction was observed in our study two weeks after the total dose of 50 U was injected into the masseter and temporal muscles bilaterally. The values were still lower 18 weeks after the drug injections, but the difference was not significant, and total recovery was achieved by 25 weeks. No significant changes in bite force were noticed after saline injections. This means that the finding of this study is due to the drug itself and not to the placebo or intervention. In a previous study using 100 U for the masseter muscles (50 U each), bite force decreased approximately 40% three months after the injections, and the values were still decreased by approximately 35% six months after the treatment [19]. Jadhau et al. also reported the lowest decrease three months after injections with 100 U of BoNT-A, the values being still lower six months later [20]. Combining these results with ours might suggest that the decreased bite force, as well as recovery rate, are dose-dependent. In a study using 42 U for the masseter muscles (21 U each) a decrease of approximately 50% was observed 10 days after the injections, with a significant reduction still present 20 weeks after the treatment [21]. Obviously, as with EMG activity, BoNT-A injection decreases bite force according to any research. However, the differences in the injection areas, doses, and timing of follow-up visits mean that the results are not directly comparable.

It is known that decreased muscle-derived force and muscle activity cause bone loss [22]. Changes in bone volume and density are also reported in studies that evaluate the effect of BoNT-A injections [12,23]. The decreased values of EMG and bite force reported in this study may predict the presence of latent adverse effects beyond the injected muscle. Alongside the mechanical theory, biochemical interactions between muscle and bone tissue have recently been the subject of interest [24]. The masticatory system, which is made up of bones, joints, ligaments, teeth, and muscles, is a highly refined unit. There is complex molecular crosstalk between components and altering the function of one component may lead to the malfunction of another component. The biomechanical and biochemical interactions are particularly important in the development phase of masticatory structures, meaning that the injections are contraindicated in growing individuals.

In our study, most patients were female (82.5%), which is partly explained by the fact that TMD is more prevalent in women than in men [25,26]. Of the sixty-six randomized patients, nine dropped out during the study. An interesting fact is that all those who left the study voluntarily received saline first and did not wait for the BoNT-A injection. This might be explained by patients' expectations of a quick fix when seeking medical help and not deriving benefit from the placebo. The high education level of the subjects of our research might reflect the patient's financial situation and thus the possibility of applying for private dental care. However, the results of the previous studies regarding associations between TMD and education level are not conclusive [27,28].

The randomization, blinding, and placebo control used in our study are gold standards to evaluate the effects of medical intervention. To reduce the heterogeneity of the subjects included in the study, a standardized examination protocol of TMD-patients (DC/TMD), as well as history and anamnesis questionnaires, were used. However, because of the randomization, the differences in the initial scores between groups could not be avoided. In this research, the initial EMGmax values were higher in the BS group than in the SB group, which, however, has no influence when the values are compared within one group.

The results reported herein should be considered in light of some limitations. First, the recovery rate reported based on the BS group findings only might be influenced by the saline injections that were performed at the 16-week follow-up. However, changes caused by saline compared to changes caused by BoNT-A, were rather insignificant, as was seen in the SB group. Second, the decreased muscle activity and bite force hardly reflect the beneficial gain of the treatment. The analgesic effect of BoNT-A is thought to be the main mechanism of action when treating pain conditions and is independent of its neuromuscular effect [17]. Masticatory muscle pain is related more to patient psychological status than muscle activity [29]. There is also evidence that occlusal forces do not correlate with TMD symptoms [30]. The findings of this research do not give information on BoNT-A indications when treating pain symptoms. While the decision to inject is always made according to the symptoms and diagnosis, there is still no consensus on the indications and dose appropriateness. Earlier studies, with doses ranging from 80 to 200 U, proved that BoNT-A's pain-relieving effect can last up to 4–6 months [5,6,16]. Up to six months of analgesic effect from BoNT-A had also been observed in the treatment of trigeminal neuralgia [31]. De Lima et al. studied the effect of 20 U on TMD pain findings, concluding that a low dose can be effective for controlling chronic pain, but this outcome was short-lived, with pain scores reaching the baseline within 30 days [32]. Whether a total dose of 50 U can be an optimal one with acceptable adverse effects in relation to therapeutic benefit remains a subject of interest. Third, even though BoNT-A injections impair skeletal muscle function, the clinical importance of this is still unclear. Side effects should be evaluated after multiple treatments with longer follow-up periods. So far, low doses of BoNT-A are suggested to be safer because the degree and duration of the adverse effects are dose-dependent [16]. In addition, according to some studies, bigger doses are not likely to bring more therapeutic benefits when treating pain conditions [16,33]. In further clinical trials, the beneficial effect of a moderate dose of BoNT-A, such as 50 U, should be evaluated.

4. Conclusions

We conclude that the recovery of muscle function occurs 33 weeks after the injection of 50 U of BoNT-A when treating masticatory muscle pain disorder. Thus, that period can be considered safe for reinjections. Further studies should evaluate the effect of this dose of the drug on pain findings and its ratio to adverse effects.

5. Materials and Methods

5.1. Patients

Voluntary subjects from several mainly private dental practices were recruited between May 2019 and April 2021. Patients could sign up for the study based on their own assessment of the need for treatment of orofacial pain, regardless of whether the condition had previously been treated conservatively or not. They were subsequently screened for specific inclusion and exclusion criteria. The total number of participants included in the study was 57, predominantly female. The inclusion criteria were age > 18, diagnosis of myalgia, myofascial pain, or headache attributable to TMD according to Diagnostic Criteria for Temporomandibular Disorders (DC/TMD) with persistent or bothersome recurrent pain for at least a year and present during the past month. The history questionnaire of the Research Diagnostic Criteria for Temporomandibular Disorders (RDC/TMD) was used to evaluate pain chronicity and frequency. Most of the patients had undergone conservative TMD treatment such as an occlusal splint or physiotherapy but without complete relief of symptoms. Exclusion criteria for the study were the following: previous injections of BoNT-A for the treatment of TMD, arthrosis, arthritis, neuromuscular pathologies, major psychiatric disorders, pregnancy, and lactation. After the end of the study, the patient's treatment was continued in accordance with Finnish Current Care Guidelines for TMD [34].

5.2. Experimental Protocol

This study was conducted as a crossover trial. Participants were randomly divided into two groups following simple randomization procedures: one which received BoNT-A first (the BS group) and the other which received saline first (the SB group). The second injection was performed after the washout period of 4 months (Figure 1). The patients were told they would receive both saline and BoNT-A once, but the order of the injections was unknown to them and the examiners. A random number table was used to allocate the participants. Randomization was performed by an investigator with no clinical involvement in the trial. Insulin syringes were filled either with BoNT-A dissolved in saline or saline only. The examiners received filled syringes marked with the code only. All syringes were similar in appearance. The codes of the substance injected were decoded and the data collected was analyzed using the patient's ID once the clinical part of the research was over.

Three examiners enrolled the participants and assigned them to interventions. The same examiners conducted the clinical part of the study including injections, patient examination, and measurements. The examiners were taught the injection techniques by a maxillofacial surgeon experienced in injections. In accordance with the DC/TMD guidelines, the competence of the examiners is level two, which includes a two-day course on the use of the DC/TMD examination protocol. They were also instructed in using the EMG and bite force measurement devices by a person who used them in previous research [35,36].

The study lasted for 8 months for each subject and included seven follow-up visits. There were 28 patients in the BS group and 29 in the SB group (Figure 1). Follow-ups were performed at 2, 11, and 16 weeks after the first injection and the second injection, respectively (i.e., 18, 27, and 32 weeks after the first injection). EMG activity and bite force measurements were evaluated at baseline and each follow-up.

5.3. Injections

The injections were performed according to the techniques reported in previous research [13,37]. Each patient received a once-off treatment of 50 units of BoNT-A (Xeomin®, supplied by Merz Pharmaceuticals GmbH, Frankfurt, Germany). The powder was dissolved in 1.5 mL of sterile saline water. In total, 2/3 of the dose was injected into the bilateral masseter muscle (16.7 units each) and 1/3 into the bilateral temporalis muscle (8.3 units each). Three injections located 1–1.5 cm apart were applied along the inferior border of the masseter, and two injections located 2 cm apart were applied along the anterior part of the temporalis. In the placebo group, 1.5 mL of saline was injected.

5.4. Treatment Outcomes

EMG and bite force measurements were performed with equipment that demonstrated reliability and repeatability in previous studies [35–37]. The examination was conducted in the same space and under the same conditions. Patients were in a sitting position, with the head supported and the Frankfort level parallel to the floor. On the intervention days, the measurements had been performed before the injections.

EMG parameters were assessed using a portable EMG device (ME 6000 recorder, Mega Electronics, Kuopio, Finland). The surface electrodes were positioned according to the anatomical landmarks on the masseter muscles. Inter-electrode distance recommendations of 30 mm were observed. The ground electrodes were placed on the chin. All electrode sites were cleaned by swabbing with 96% alcohol. For the analysis, the averaged EMG spectrum area data values calculated from a 2 s period were used.

Bite force was recorded with a device based on a quartz force transducer as a sensor. The sensor was built inside the 10 mm thick steel housing which was inserted along the dental arch so that the sensor was in the first molar region on the right site. To protect the teeth, the housing was covered with 2-mm-thick rubber plates on both sites. The maximal bite force value (N) could be seen on the screen of the bite force recorder.

Bilateral masseter muscle EMG activities and bite force were assessed in two serial recordings. A series of recordings consisted of a 30 s long exercise so that once every 10 s the patient should bite hard for 5 s following a 5 s relaxation. The total time of the recordings was 60 s with a few minutes break between the series. The patient was able to view the timing of the task on a computer screen. The EMGrest value used in the analysis was picked from the beginning of the recording. The EMGmax value used in the analysis was picked from the middle of the first series. The average of three maximal bite force measurements during a 60 s recording was calculated and used in the analysis.

5.5. Statistical Analysis

Parameters for power sample size estimation were determined by the authors as follows: test power 0.90 with a 0.05 significance level and effect size of 0.4. Considering these parameters, the appropriate sample size would have been 15 subjects. Other analyses of the research material and 50% dropout risk were also taken into account. Under these circumstances, the authors decided to recruit 120 subjects for the study in the first place. In the data used in this study, the observed test power was 1.0 with a significance level of <0.001 and an effect size of 0.51.

Mean values of EMG and bite force were calculated for each follow-up time. p-values were calculated for dependent mean variables using the Wilcoxon signed-rank test. Analyses were performed using SPSS version 28.0 (SPSS Inc., Chicago, IL, USA) and Office 365 Excel software 2108 (Microsoft Inc., Redmond, WA, USA).

Author Contributions: Conceptualization, V.S. and A.K.; methodology P.K. and O.T.; formal analysis, A.K.; investigation, V.S.; resources, P.K. and O.T.; data curation, V.S.; writing—original draft preparation, V.S. and A.K.; writing—review and editing, P.K. and O.T.; visualization, V.S. and A.K.; supervision, V.S.; project administration, V.S. All authors have read and agreed to the published version of the manuscript.

Funding: This research received no external funding.

Institutional Review Board Statement: The study adhered to the tenets of the Declaration of Helsinki and the regional Ethics Review Board of Helsinki University Hospital approved the study protocol (ID: HUS/3167/2018, date: 12 May 2018).

Informed Consent Statement: Informed consent was obtained from all subjects involved in the study.

Data Availability Statement: Data are available upon reasonable request.

Acknowledgments: Merz Pharmaceutical GmbH is acknowledged for providing the botulinum toxin used in this study. Open access funding provided by University of Helsinki.

Conflicts of Interest: The authors declare no conflict of interest.

References

1. Manfredini, D.; Ahlberg, J.; Winocur, E.; Guarda-Nardini, L.; Lobbezoo, F. Correlation of RDC/TMD axis I diagnoses and axis II pain-related disability. A multicenter study. *Clin. Oral Investig.* **2011**, *15*, 749–756. [CrossRef] [PubMed]
2. Ananthan, S.; Benoliel, R. Chronic orofacial pain. *J. Neural Transm.* **2020**, *127*, 575–588. [CrossRef] [PubMed]
3. Fricton, J.R. The relationship of temporomandibular disorders and fibromyalgia: Implications for diagnosis and treatment. *Curr. Pain Headache Rep.* **2004**, *8*, 355–363. [CrossRef] [PubMed]
4. Ernberg, M.; Hedenberg-Magnusson, B.; List, T.; Svensson, P. Efficacy of botulinum toxin type A for treatment of persistent myofascial TMD pain: A randomized, controlled, double-blind multicenter study. *Pain* **2011**, *152*, 1988–1996. [CrossRef] [PubMed]
5. Guarda-Nardini, L.; Stecco, A.; Stecco, C.; Masiero, S.; Manfredini, D. Myofascial pain of the jaw muscles: Comparison of short-term effectiveness of botulinum toxin injections and fascial manipulation technique. *Cranio* **2012**, *30*, 95–102. [CrossRef] [PubMed]
6. Patel, A.A.; Lerner, M.Z.; Blitzer, A. IncobotulinumtoxinA Injection for Temporomandibular Joint Disorder. *Ann. Otol. Rhinol. Laryngol.* **2017**, *126*, 328–333. [CrossRef]
7. De la Torre Canales, G.; Poluha, R.L.; Lora, V.M.; Araújo Oliveira Ferreira, D.M.; Stuginski-Barbosa, J.; Bonjardim, L.R.; Cury, A.A.D.B.; Conti, P.C.R. Botulinum toxin type A applications for masticatory myofascial pain and trigeminal neuralgia: What is the evidence regarding adverse effects? *Clin. Oral Investig.* **2019**, *23*, 3411–3421. [CrossRef]
8. la Fleur, P.; Adams, A. *Botulinum Toxin for Temporomandibular Disorders: A Review of Clinical Effectiveness, Cost-Effectiveness, and Guidelines [Internet]*; Canadian Agency for Drugs and Technologies in Health: Ottawa, ON, Canada, 2020.
9. Serrera-Figallo, M.A.; Ruiz-de-León-Hernández, G.; Torres-Lagares, D.; Castro-Araya, A.; Torres-Ferrerosa, O.; Hernández-Pacheco, E.; Gutierrez-Perez, J.L. Use of Botulinum Toxin in Orofacial Clinical Practice. *Toxins* **2020**, *12*, 112. [CrossRef]
10. Yamauchi, P.S.; Lowe, N.J. Botulinum toxin types A and B: Comparison of efficacy, duration, and dose-ranging studies for the treatment of facial rhytides and hyperhidrosis. *Clin. Dermatol.* **2004**, *22*, 34–39. [CrossRef]
11. Lee, C.J.; Kim, S.G.; Kim, Y.J.; Han, J.Y.; Choi, S.H.; Lee, S.I. Electrophysiologic change and facial contour following botulinum toxin A injection in square faces. *Plast. Reconstr. Surg.* **2007**, *120*, 769–778. [CrossRef]
12. Balanta-Melo, J.; Toro-Ibacache, V.; Kupczik, K.; Buvinic, S. Mandibular Bone Loss after Masticatory Muscles Intervention with Botulinum Toxin: An Approach from Basic Research to Clinical Findings. *Toxins* **2019**, *11*, 84. [CrossRef] [PubMed]
13. Kahn, A.; Kün-Darbois, J.D.; Bertin, H.; Corre, P.; Chappard, D. Mandibular bone effects of botulinum toxin injections in masticatory muscles in adult. *Oral Surg. Oral Med. Oral Pathol. Oral Radiol.* **2020**, *129*, 100–108. [CrossRef] [PubMed]
14. Baldwin, M.C.; Liu, Z.J.; Rafferty, K.L.; Keith, A.; Tamasas, B.; Kaiyala, K.; Herring, S.W. Botulinum toxin in the masseter muscle: Lingering effects of denervation. *Anat. Rec.* **2022**, *305*, 1215–1230. [CrossRef]
15. Kim, N.H.; Park, R.H.; Park, J.B. Botulinum toxin type A for the treatment of hypertrophy of the masseter muscle. *Plast. Reconstr. Surg.* **2010**, *125*, 1693–1705. [CrossRef]
16. De la Torre Canales, G.; Alvarez-Pinzon, N.; Muñoz-Lora, V.R.M.; Vieira Peroni, L.; Farias Gomes, A.; Sánchez-Ayala, A.; Haiter-Neto, F.; Manfredini, D.; Rizzatti-Barbosa, C.M. Efficacy and Safety of Botulinum Toxin Type A on Persistent Myofascial Pain: A Randomized Clinical Trial. *Toxins* **2020**, *12*, 395. [CrossRef] [PubMed]
17. De La Torre Canales, G.; Câmara-Souza, M.B.; Poluha, R.L.; Grillo, C.M.; Conti, P.C.R.; Sousa, M.D.L.R.; Rodrigues Garcia, R.C.M.; Rizzatti-Barbosa, C.M. Botulinum toxin type A and acupuncture for masticatory myofascial pain: A randomized clinical trial. *J. Appl. Oral Sci.* **2021**, *29*, e20201035. [CrossRef] [PubMed]
18. Kurtoglu, C.; Gur, O.H.; Kurkcu, M.; Sertdemir, Y.; Guler-Uysal, F.; Uysal, H. Effect of botulinum toxin-A in myofascial pain patients with or without functional disc displacement. *J. Oral Maxillofac. Surg.* **2008**, *66*, 1644–1651. [CrossRef]
19. Zhang, L.D.; Liu, Q.; Zou, D.R.; Yu, L.F. Occlusal force characteristics of masseteric muscles after intramuscular injection of botulinum toxin A(BTX—A)for treatment of temporomandibular disorder. *Br. J. Oral Maxillofac. Surg.* **2016**, *54*, 736–740. [CrossRef]
20. Jadhao, V.A.; Lokhande, N.; Habbu, S.G.; Sewane, S.; Dongare, S.; Goyal, N. Efficacy of botulinum toxin in treating myofascial pain and occlusal force characteristics of masticatory muscles in bruxism. *Indian J. Dent. Res.* **2017**, *28*, 493–497. [CrossRef]

21. Pihut, M.; Wisniewska, G.; Majewski, P.; Gronkiewicz, K.; Majewski, S. Measurement of occlusal forces in the therapy of functional disorders with the use of botulinum toxin type A. *J. Physiol. Pharmacol.* **2009**, *60* (Suppl. 8), 113–116.
22. Bettis, T.; Kim, B.J.; Hamrick, M.W. Impact of muscle atrophy on bone metabolism and bone strength: Implications for muscle-bone crosstalk with aging and disuse. *Osteoporos. Int.* **2018**, *29*, 1713–1720. [CrossRef] [PubMed]
23. Raphael, K.G.; Tadinada, A.; Bradshaw, J.M.; Janal, M.N.; Sirois, D.A.; Chan, K.C.; Lurie, A.G. Osteopenic consequences of botulinum toxin injections in the masticatory muscles: A pilot study. *J. Oral Rehabil.* **2014**, *41*, 555–563. [CrossRef]
24. Buvinic, S.; Balanta-Melo, J.; Kupczik, K.; Vásquez, W.; Beato, C.; Toro-Ibacache, V. Muscle-Bone Crosstalk in the Masticatory System: From Biomechanical to Molecular Interactions. *Front. Endocrinol.* **2021**, *11*, 606947. [CrossRef]
25. Bueno, C.H.; Pereira, D.D.; Pattussi, M.P.; Grossi, P.K.; Grossi, M.L. Gender differences in temporomandibular disorders in adult populational studies: A systematic review and meta-analysis. *J. Oral Rehabil.* **2018**, *45*, 720–729. [CrossRef]
26. Johansson, A.; Unell, L.; Carlsson, G.E.; Söderfeldt, B.; Halling, A. Gender difference in symptoms related to temporomandibular disorders in a population of 50-year-old subjects. *J. Orofac. Pain* **2003**, *17*, 29–35. [PubMed]
27. Yekkalam, N.; Wänman, A. Associations between craniomandibular disorders, sociodemographic factors and self-perceived general and oral health in an adult population. *Acta Odontol. Scand.* **2014**, *72*, 1054–1065. [CrossRef] [PubMed]
28. Macfarlane, T.V.; Glenny, A.M.; Worthington, H.V. Systematic review of population-based epidemiological studies of orofacial pain. *J. Dent.* **2001**, *29*, 451–467. [CrossRef]
29. van Selms, M.K.; Lobbezoo, F.; Visscher, C.M.; Naeije, M. Myofascial temporomandibular disorder pain, parafunctions and psychological stress. *J. Oral Rehabil.* **2008**, *35*, 45–52. [CrossRef]
30. Ahlberg, J.P.; Kovero, O.A.; Hurmerinta, K.A.; Zepa, I.; Nissinen, M.J.; Könönen, M.H. Maximal bite force and its association with signs and symptoms of TMD, occlusion, and body mass index in a cohort of young adults. *Cranio* **2003**, *21*, 248–252. [CrossRef]
31. Zhang, H.; Lian, Y.; Xie, N.; Chen, C.; Zheng, Y. Single-dose botulinum toxin type a compared with repeated-dose for treatment of trigeminal neuralgia: A pilot study. *J. Headache Pain* **2017**, *18*, 81. [CrossRef]
32. de Lima, M.C.; Rizzatti Barbosa, C.M.; Duarte Gavião, M.B.; Ferreira Caria, P.H. Is low dose of botulinum toxin effective in controlling chronic pain in sleep bruxism, awake bruxism, and temporomandibular disorder? *Cranio* **2021**, *6*, 1–8. [CrossRef] [PubMed]
33. Zhang, H.; Lian, Y.; Ma, Y.; Chen, Y.; He, C.; Xie, N.; Wu, C. Two doses of botulinum toxin type A for the treatment of trigeminal neuralgia: Observation of therapeutic effect from a randomized, double-blind, placebo-controlled trial. *J. Headache Pain* **2014**, *15*, 65. [CrossRef] [PubMed]
34. Purentaelimistön kipu ja toimintahäiriöt (TMD). *Current Care Guidelines. Working Group Set up by the Finnish Medical Society Duodecim and the Finnish Dental Society Apollonia*; The Finnish Medical Society Duodecim: Helsinki, Finland, 2021.
35. Kemppainen, P.; Waltimo, A.; Waltimo, T.; Könönen, M.; Pertovaara, A. Differential effects of noxious conditioning stimulation of the cheek by capsaicin on human sensory and inhibitory masseter reflex responses evoked by tooth pulp stimulation. *J. Dent. Res.* **1997**, *76*, 1561–1568. [CrossRef]
36. Suvinen, T.I.; Malmberg, J.; Forster, C.; Kemppainen, P. Postural and dynamic masseter and anterior temporalis muscle EMG repeatability in serial assessments. *J. Oral Rehabil.* **2009**, *36*, 814–820. [CrossRef] [PubMed]
37. Sitnikova, V.; Kämppi, A.; Teronen, O.; Kemppainen, P. Comprehensive evaluation of botulinum toxin treatment outcomes of a patient with persistent myofascial orofacial pain. *Clin. Case Rep.* **2021**, *9*, e04731. [CrossRef] [PubMed]

toxins

MDPI

Article

Efficacy of Botulinum Toxin Type-A I in the Improvement of Mandibular Motion and Muscle Sensibility in Myofascial Pain TMD Subjects: A Randomized Controlled Trial

Giancarlo De la Torre Canales [1,2,*], Rodrigo Lorenzi Poluha [3], Natalia Alvarez Pinzón [4], Bruno Rodrigues Da Silva [5], Andre Mariz Almeida [1], Malin Ernberg [6], Ana Cristina Manso [1], Leonardo Rigoldi Bonjardim [7] and Célia Marisa Rizzatti-Barbosa [2]

1 Clinical Research Unit (CRU), Centro de Investigação Interdisciplinar Egas Moniz (CiiEM), Egas Moniz—Cooperativa de Ensino Superior, CRL, Quinta da Granja, Monte de Caparica, 2829-511 Caparica, Portugal; andremarizalmeida@gmail.com (A.M.A.); mansocristina@gmail.com (A.C.M.)
2 Ingá University Center, Uningá, Maringa 87020-900, Brazil; rizzatti@unicamp.br
3 Department of Dentistry, State University of Maringa, Maringa 87020-900, Brazil; rodrigopoluha@gmail.com
4 Institución Universitaria Colegios de Colombia-Centro de Investigación del Colegio Odontológico (CICO) 20, Bogotá 111611, Colombia; natalialvarezodont@gmail.com
5 Private Practice—Boavista Avenue, 4100-139 Porto, Portugal; brunomrsb@hotmail.com
6 Department of Dental Medicine, Karolinska Institutet, and the Scandinavian Center for Orofacial Neurosciences (SCON), 141 52 Huddinge, Sweden; malin.ernberg@ki.se
7 Bauru Orofacial Pain Group, Department of Biological Sciences, Bauru School of Dentistry, University of São Paulo, Sao Paulo 17012-900, Brazil; lbonjardim@fob.usp.br
* Correspondence: giank_28@hotmail.com

Citation: De la Torre Canales, G.; Poluha, R.L.; Pinzón, N.A.; Da Silva, B.R.; Almeida, A.M.; Ernberg, M.; Manso, A.C.; Bonjardim, L.R.; Rizzatti-Barbosa, C.M. Efficacy of Botulinum Toxin Type-A I in the Improvement of Mandibular Motion and Muscle Sensibility in Myofascial Pain TMD Subjects: A Randomized Controlled Trial. *Toxins* **2022**, *14*, 441. https://doi.org/10.3390/toxins14070441

Received: 3 June 2022
Accepted: 24 June 2022
Published: 29 June 2022

Abstract: This study assessed the effects of botulinum toxin type A (BoNT-A) in mandibular range of motion and muscle tenderness to palpation in persistent myofascial pain (MFP) patients (ReBEC RBR-2d4vvv). Eighty consecutive female subjects with persistent MFP, were randomly divided into four groups ($n = 20$): three BoNT-A groups with different doses and a saline solution group (placebo control group). Treatments were injected bilaterally in the masseter and anterior temporalis muscle in a single session. Clinical measurements of mandibular movements included: pain-free opening, maximum unassisted and assisted opening, and right and left lateral excursions. Palpation tests were performed bilaterally in the masseter and temporalis muscle. Follow-up occurred 28 and 180 days after treatment. For the statistical analysis the Mann–Whitney U-test with Bonferroni correction was used for groups comparisons. Regardless of dose, all parameters of mandibular range of motion significantly improved after 180 days in all BoNT-A groups, compared with the control group. Palpation pain over the masseter and temporalis muscles were significantly reduced in all BoNT-A groups regardless of dose, compared with the control group, after 28 and 180 days of treatment. Independent of doses, BoNT-A improved mandibular range of motion and muscle tenderness to palpation in persistent MFP patients.

Keywords: botulinum toxin type A; myofascial pain; temporomandibular disorders

Key Contribution: Botulinum toxin could be a therapeutic option for patients that do not get substantial relieve from common-conservative treatments. Its beneficial effects on muscle pain and mandibular movements are not doses dependent.

1. Introduction

Temporomandibular disorders (TMDs) are a heterogeneous group of conditions that affect the masticatory muscles, temporomandibular joint, and associated structures [1]. Myofascial pain (MFP) is one of the most observed TMDs diagnoses, affecting 38% to 75% of the Caucasian population and around 30% of the Asiatic population, and represents 45%

of subject with TMD [2]. This condition is defined as a regional muscle pain associated with tenderness to palpation [3] and is most prevalent in young and middle-aged adults (mean age of 30–40 years) and with a higher prevalence in females [2]. The clinical presentation of MFP includes pain referral, tenderness, or pain at the site of palpation, and restriction in the range of motion.

The Research Diagnostic Criteria for TMD (RDC/TMD) [3] and its updated version the Diagnostic Criteria for TMD (DC/TMD) [4] are the most used instruments for TMD diagnoses. They are constituted by a dual-axis system: Axis I, based on the medical history of clinical conditions and Axis II which focuses on pain related disability and psychosocial status assessment [5]. The Axis I protocol is a standardized series of diagnostic tests based on clinical signs and symptoms relying on the outcomes of palpation tests and mandibular range of motion as important findings for diagnostic purposes [3]. Therefore, using the Axis I clinical parameters to assess the outcomes of an MFP treatment in muscle sensitivity and mandibular movements is extremely important in clinical practice and brings reliable data.

Considering the favorable course of TMDs including MFP [6], conservative and reversible treatments (e.g., occlusal splints, behavioral therapies, needling techniques, laser therapy, pharmacotherapy, and physiotherapy) are preferable to more aggressive and irreversible approaches in the initial treatment of MFP since they are effective in reducing painful symptoms [7–10]. Notwithstanding, the complex etiopathogenesis of MFP [11] make that the use of these conventional and minimally invasive therapies as first line treatment is not enough in some cases [12]. Then, new treatment approaches such as botulinum toxin type A (BoNT-A) are proposed with a promising potential to diminish pain [13]. In addition, since the US-FDA approved BoNT-A as a treatment for many muscle and pain disorders [14], animal studies have showed that BoNT-A have analgesic effects and inhibits nociceptive mediators release (peripherally and centrally), a mechanism separate of its neuromotor effect.

According to the American Academy of Neurology, BoNT-A is classified as a level B treatment (possibly effective) for MFP [15]. However, literature is still not clear about the efficacy of BoNT-A in the improvement of MFP, since well-designed clinical trials presented opposite results when compared BoNT-A with a placebo, and not demonstrated the superiority of BoNT-A over classic treatments like oral appliances [16]. Flaws like the lack of standardized protocols of application and a proper methodological design, contribute to this lack of consensus [16]. Additionally, even though BoNT-A treatment is considered generally safe, a recent systematic review concluded that BoNTA injection could results in mandibular bony change, which may hinder BoNT-A benefits [17].

Based on the conflicting results available on the use of BoNT-A for MFP, it is im-portant to assess treatment effect on other parameters besides pain intensity in patients with MFP. Especially since this toxin may have a use as an alternative in cases where the conventional treatments fail. Thus, the aim of this randomized, placebo controlled clinical trial was to demonstrate the efficacy of BoNT-A in the improvement of mandibular range of motion and muscle sensibility to palpation in persistent MFP patients.

2. Results

2.1. Subjects

Eighty consecutive female subjects, who were diagnosed with MFP, according to the Brazilian Portuguese version of the RDC/TMD [3] at the TMD Clinic of Piracicaba Dental School, University of Campinas, São Paulo, Brazil, were included. Subjects were assessed by two calibrated researchers not involved in any other process of the study (kappa coefficient = 0.80 for RDC/TMD inter-examiner assessment).

2.2. Mandibular Motion

Considering the pain-free mouth opening, there was no difference between groups at baseline and at the 28 days follow-up ($p > 0.05$), and no changes within groups during the first month ($p > 0.05$) of follow-up (Table 1). However, at the 180-day evaluation, all

BoNT-A groups showed a significant improvement compared with the other evaluation periods ($p < 0.05$). In contrast, a decrease in pain-free mouth opening was found in the SS group. In the between group comparisons, all BoNT-A groups presented a greater increase ($p < 0.05$) in pain-free mouth opening compared with the control group at the 180-day evaluation (Table 1).

Table 1. Mean and standard deviation of pain-free opening (mm) in different evaluation periods.

	Time					
	Baseline		28 Days		180 Days	
Groups	Mean	SD	Mean	SD	Mean	SD
BoNTA-L	31.9 aB	8.7	33.6 aB	8.8	38.3 aA	7.5
BoNTA-M	32.4 aB	9.4	35.0 aB	7.7	40.7 aA	7.6
BoNTA-H	32.6 aB	8.9	35.0 aB	9.2	39.0 aA	8.1
SS	36.2 aB	6.1	37.6 aB	6.6	34.0 bA	9.0

Different letters (lowercase in vertical) represent significant difference ($p \leq 0.05$) among groups. Different letters (uppercase in horizontal) represent significant difference ($p \leq 0.05$) among evaluation periods. BoNTA: botulinum toxin type A; L: low; M: median; H: high; SS: saline solution; SD: standard deviation.

The same pattern was observed for maximum unassisted and assisted mouth opening (Table 2). A significant improvement was found at the 180-day follow-up only in the BoNT-A groups. Moreover, the groups showed higher unassisted and assisted mouth opening in the BoNT-A groups compared with SS ($p < 0.05$) at the last follow-up (Table 2).

Table 2. Median, minimum, and maximum values for maximum unassisted and assisted opening in different evaluation periods.

		Time								
		Baseline			28 Days			180 Days		
	Groups	Median	Mn	Mx	Median	Mn	Mx	Median	Mn	Mx
Unassisted	BoNTA-L	41.0 aB	28.0	59.0	42.0 aB	29.0	58.0	44.5 aA	31.0	60.0
	BoNTA-M	43.0 aB	29.0	54.0	43.5 aB	30.0	52.0	45.0 aA	35.0	60.0
	BoNTA-H	41.0 aB	26.0	50.0	43.0 aB	25.0	52.0	46.0 aA	23.0	55.0
	SS	41.5 aB	35.0	55.0	42.0 aB	50.0	50.0	39.0 bB	20.0	45.0
Assisted	BoNTA-L	43.0 aB	30.0	60.0	43.0 aB	31.0	58.0	47.0 aA	33.0	62.0
	BoNTA-M	47.0 aB	30.0	57.0	45.5 aB	31.0	55.0	48.5 aA	35.0	61.0
	BoNTA-H	44.0 aB	30.0	55.0	47.0 aB	30.0	53.0	50.0 aA	31.0	57.0
	SS	42.5 aB	33.0	56.0	43.5 aB	34.0	51.0	41.5 bB	22.0	47.0

Different letters (lowercase in vertical) represent significant difference ($p \leq 0.05$) among groups. Different letters (uppercase in horizontal) represent significant difference ($p \leq 0.05$) among evaluation periods. BoNTA: botulinum toxin type A; L: low; M: median; H: high; SS: Saline Solution. Mn: minimum; Mx: maximum.

Regarding right and left lateral movements, no significant differences were found in the group comparisons at baseline and after 28 days of treatment ($p < 0.05$). However, in the 180-day evaluation the BoNT-A groups showed a significant increase in all lateral movements ($p < 0.05$) without significant differences among them. In contrast, no significant differences were found in the SS group in any period of evaluation. Furthermore, BoNT-A groups showed higher values at the 180-day follow-up ($p < 0.05$) compared with the SS group (Table 3).

2.3. Muscle Pain

Considering the mean of pain on palpation in masseter and temporalis muscles of both sides (Tables 4 and 5), the BoNT-A groups reported significantly reduced pain sensbility to palpation at the 28-day follow-up ($p < 0.05$). This significant improvement remained until the 180-day evaluation ($p < 0.05$), but without differences between BoNT-A groups

($p > 0.05$). The SS group showed no significant differences in any period of assessment ($p > 0.05$). Comparisons between BoNT-A and SS showed lower values for BoNT-A groups at the 28- and 180-day follow-ups ($p < 0.05$).

Table 3. Median, minimum, and maximum values for right and left lateral movements in different evaluation periods.

		Time								
		Baseline			28 Days			180 Days		
	Groups	**Median**	**Mn**	**Mx**	**Median**	**Mn**	**Mx**	**Median**	**Mn**	**Mx**
Right	BoNTA-L	9.5 aA	2.0	15.0	9.0 aA	3.0	12.0	11.0 aB	6.0	13.0
	BoNTA-M	9.0 aA	5.0	12.0	9.0 aA	6.0	14.0	10.0 aB	7.0	13.0
	BoNTA-H	8.5 aA	4.0	14.0	9.5 aA	4.0	14.0	10.5 aB	5.0	15.0
	SS	8.0 aA	3.0	11.0	8.5 aA	5.0	14.0	9.0 bA	5.0	12.0
Left	BoNTA-L	8.0 aA	0.0	13.0	9.0 aA	4.0	13.0	9.5 aB	4.0	14.0
	BoNTA-M	8.0 aA	2.0	12.0	9.0 aA	6.0	15.0	10.0 aB	8.0	15.0
	BoNTA-H	9.5 aA	4.0	12.0	9.5 aA	4.0	15.0	10.0 aB	6.0	15.0
	SS	8.0 aA	3.0	13.0	8.5 aA	5.0	15.0	8.5 bA	5.0	15.0

Different letters (lowercase in vertical) represent significant difference ($p \leq 0.05$) among groups. Different letters (uppercase in horizontal) represent significant difference ($p \leq 0.05$) among evaluation periods. BoNTA: botulinum toxin type A; L: low; M: median; H: high; SS: Saline Solution. Mn: minimum; Mx: maximum.

Table 4. Median, minimum, and maximum values for right and left masseter muscle in different evaluation periods.

		Time								
		Baseline			28 Days			180 Days		
	Groups	**Median**	**Mn**	**Mx**	**Median**	**Mn**	**Mx**	**Median**	**Mn**	**Mx**
Right	BoNTA-L	2.0 aA	0.0	3.0	1.0 bB	0.0	12.0	0.5 bB	0.0	2.0
	BoNTA-M	1.0 aA	0.0	3.0	0.0 bB	0.0	14.0	0.0 bB	0.0	3.0
	BoNTA-H	2.0 aA	0.0	3.0	0.5 bB	0.0	14.0	0.0 bB	0.0	3.0
	SS	2.0 aA	1.0	3.0	2.0 aA	0.0	14.0	2.0 aA	0.0	3.0
Left	BoNTA-L	1.5 aA	0.0	3.0	0.0 bB	0.0	2.0	0.5 bB	0.0	3.0
	BoNTA-M	1.0 aA	0.0	3.0	0.0 bB	0.0	3.0	0.0 bB	0.0	3.0
	BoNTA-H	2.0 aA	0.0	3.0	0.0 bB	0.0	3.0	0.0 bB	0.0	2.0
	SS	1.0 aA	0.0	3.0	2.0 aA	0.0	3.0	2.0 aA	0.0	3.0

Different letters (lowercase in vertical) represent significant difference ($p \leq 0.05$) among groups. Different letters (uppercase in horizontal) represent significant difference ($p \leq 0.05$) evaluation periods. BoNTA: botulinum toxin type A; L: low; M: median; H: high; SS: Saline Solution. Mn: minimum; Mx: maximum.

Table 5. Median, minimum, and maximum values for right and left temporal muscle in different evaluation periods.

		Time								
		Baseline			28 Days			180 Days		
	Groups	**Median**	**Mn**	**Mx**	**Median**	**Mn**	**Mx**	**Median**	**Mn**	**Mx**
Right	BoNTA-L	2.5 aA	0.0	3.0	1.0 bB	0.0	2.0	0.0 aB	0.0	2.0
	BoNTA-M	2.0 aA	0.0	3.0	1.0 bB	0.0	2.0	0.0 aB	0.0	2.0
	BoNTA-H	2.0 aA	0.0	3.0	0.0 bB	0.0	3.0	0.5 aB	0.0	2.0
	SS	2.0 aA	0.0	3.0	2.0 aA	0.0	3.0	2.0 bA	0.0	3.0
Left	BoNTA-L	2.0 aA	0.0	3.0	1.0 bB	0.0	3.0	0.5 aB	0.0	2.0
	BoNTA-M	1.5 aA	0.0	3.0	0.0 bB	0.0	3.0	0.0 aB	0.0	2.0
	BoNTA-H	2.0 aA	0.0	3.0	0.5 bB	0.0	3.0	0.0 aB	0.0	2.0
	SS	1.5 aA	0.0	3.0	1.0 bA	0.0	3.0	1.5 bA	0.0	3.0

Different letters (lowercase in vertical) represent significant difference ($p \leq 0.05$) among groups. Different letters (uppercase in horizontal) represent significant difference ($p \leq 0.05$) evaluation periods. BoNTA: botulinum toxin type A; L: low; M: median; H: high; SS: Saline Solution. Mn: minimum; Mx: maximum.

3. Discussion

To the best of our knowledge, this is the first randomized, placebo-controlled clinical trial to demonstrate that independent of dosage, BoNT-A improves mandibular range of motion (pain-free opening of the mouth, maximum unassisted and assisted mouth opening, and right and left lateral mandibular movements) and muscle sensibility to palpation (in masseter and temporal muscles bilateral) in persistent MFP patients compared with a placebo.

Restriction in mandibular range of motion is one of the most common clinical presentations of MFP and usually it is used as a parameter to assess treatment efficacy. One of the most relevant results from the present study was the improvement of mandibular range of motion in persistent MFP patients treated with BoNT-A (Tables 1–3). After 180 days of treatment, all BoNT-A groups showed a significant increase in pain-free mouth opening, maximum unassisted and assisted mouth opening, and right and left lateral mandibular movements. These results corroborate available literature that also presented a gain of mandibular range of motion in MFP patients when treated with BoNT-A (100 to 150 U, distributed among masseter, temporal, and medial pterygoid muscle bilateral) compared with injections of saline solution and lidocaine [8,18]. However, since other studies such as the one performed by Ernberg et al., 2011 [19] reported no significant changes for these parameters, no definitive conclusions can be made as to whether BoNT-A injections improve mandibular range of motion. It is interesting to note that in the present study, the increase in mandibular range of motion was not influenced by the BoNT-A doses; all groups treated with BoNT-A had a greater increase compared with the control group. In fact, patients in the control group, after 180 days of follow-up, showed decreased values of pain-free mouth opening as well as unassisted and assisted mouth opening, demonstrating that SS was not effective in ameliorating these parameters.

In the research field and in every day clinical practice it is more and more evident that BoNT-A has an antinociceptive effect in muscle conditions [13,14,16]. Considering the results of our study regarding pain sensibility on palpation in masseter and temporalis muscles, BoNT-A groups showed significantly reduced pain sensitivity to palpation 28 days after treatment and this improvement remained for 180 days after treatment. The improvement in this pain parameter is in accordance with other studies where patients with persistent MFP treated with BoNT-A, presented a significant reduction in different pain measurements including the pain pressure threshold of the masticatory muscles [20–23]. Moreover, the fact that in our study, the positive effects of a single injection of BoNT-A in the assessed variables lasted for 6 months, can clinically explain that the antinociceptive effect of BoNT-A is independent of muscle paralysis which last for 3 to 4 months [24].

Taken together, the increased mandibular range of motion and the reduction in muscle sensibility to palpation found in the present study after the BoNT-A treatment, warrants some discussion. First, the improvement of all variables related to the mandibular range of motion was significant only 180 days after treatment, while a significant improvement in the muscle sensibility to palpation was observed already 28 days after treatment. These findings are understandable since it is well-known that pain can restrict movements, whether by kinesiophobia and/or muscle protective contraction [25–28]. Therefore, it is expected that the mandibular range of motion only improves after a significant reduction of muscle sensibility. If this study had a monthly follow-up of the variables, this relationship would be better elucidated. Additionally, this reasoning also serves as an alert for the importance of pain improvement as soon as possible in cases of MFP in order to obtain a quicklier improvement in mandibular movements or a reduction in movement pain. Second, even though in our study BoNT-A was only injected in the masseter and temporalis muscles, a significant improvement in the assessed mandibular movements in which other muscles such as medial and lateral pterygoid participate was also achieved. These results demonstrate that by diminishing muscle pain, BoNT-A can perhaps reestablish the equilibrium in masticatory musculature function [29,30].

Some animal and clinical studies have demonstrated that BoNT-A injections in masticatory muscles could produce adverse effects such as: alter masticatory performance, in-duce muscle atrophy, and diminish mandibular bone volume [31]. In addition, these ad-verse effects are proportional with the doses and number of applications of BoNT-A [31].

Interestingly, the positive results found in the BoNT-A groups in our study, were not ifluenced by the BoNT-A doses, showing that low doses were equally efficient as median and higher doses in improving mandibular range of motion and muscle palpation pain in patients with persistent MFP. These results are in line with our previous study comparing BoNT-A doses [32] in which pain intensity and sensibility (pain pressure threshold) were improved regardless of dosage. In addition, no adverse effects in muscle and bone tissue with low doses of BoNT-A were found in that study. Notwithstanding, in our previous study [32] a single injection of 50U and 70U and 20U and 25U in masseter and anterior temporalis muscles respectively, produced a reduction in muscles thickness and a de-crease in mandibular bone volume (coronoid process and mandibular head), showing that adverse effects are doses dependent [32]. Therefore, it could be proposed that regardless of doses, BoNT-A also diminish pain and improve mandibular movements [23] with low risks of developing serious adverse effects when low doses are used.

Nevertheless, caution is suggested when judging the present findings, since this investigation was performed on a restricted population (persistent MFP) and without gender comparison. Future studies with larger samples, using even lower doses of BoNT-A, com-paring its efficacy with other treatments are encouraged. Additionally, due to BoNT-A potential to develop adverse effects, we recommend indicating this treatment just in myofascial pain TMD patients who did not obtain a substantial pain relieve with conservative treatments.

4. Conclusions

In view of the results and limitations of this study, it can be concluded that BoNT-A, independent of dosage, improves mandibular range of motion (pain-free opening of the mouth, maximum unassisted and assisted mouth opening, and right and left lateral mandibular movements) and muscle pain to palpation of the masseter and temporal muscles in persistent MFP patients compared with SS injections.

5. Methods

The present study was approved by the Research Ethics Committee of Piracicaba Dental School (CAAE # 22953113.8.0000.5418-Date: 4 February 2014) and the Brazilian Regis-try of Clinical Trials (ReBEC RBR-2d4vvv). Subjects were recruited at the TMD Clinic of Piracicaba Dental School, University of Campinas, São Paulo, Brazil, from June 2014 to May 2017. All subjects provided a written informed consent to participate in this clinical trial This study was based on a secondary data analysis of our previous publication De la Tor-re Canales et al., 2020 [29].

5.1. Inclusion Criteria

- Years of age: 18–45;
- A diagnosis of MFP according to the RDC/TMD classification [3]
- No significant pain relief after at least three months of previous treatment;
- A baseline pain intensity of at least 50 on a visual analogue scale (VAS: 0–100);
- Subjects were also included if they presented other non-painful TMD diagnoses besides MFP.

5.2. Exclusion Criteria

- History of trauma in the face and neck area;
- Dental pain in the last 6 months;
- Systemic diseases (arthritis and arthrosis) and major psychiatric disorders;
- Current use of drugs acting on neuromuscular junctions;
- Contraindication or hypersensitivity to BoNT-A;
- Received anti-tetanus vaccine in the 3 months before the start of the clinical trial.

The sample was randomly divided into four equal groups (n = 20): BoNT-A low (BoNTA-L/10 U in each temporalis and 30 U in each masseter), BoNT-A medium (BoNTA-M/20 U in each temporalis and 50 U in each masseter), BoNT-A high (BoNTA-H/25 U in each temporalis and 75 U in each masseter), and saline solution 0.9% ((SS) placebo control group). To blind applications, each muscle received an injection containing 1 mL of the correspondent reconstituted BoNT-A-L/M/H doses or SS by a clinician not involved in the reconstitution process. Randomization was performed using a computer software (Isfahan, Iran https://random-allocation-software.software.informer.com/2.0/ (accessed on 15 November 2013) operated by a technician not involved in any other procedures in the study.

5.3. Treatments

A counseling session was performed for all the included subjects at the first appointment by a single trained researcher. In brief, counseling consisted in educating the subjects about the anatomic characteristics and physiology of the stomatognathic system and the etiology, evolution, and prognosis of MFP, teaching self-care strategies for pain and to control parafunctional habits and giving information about improvement of sleep and the importance of dietary habits.

BoNT-A (100 U; Botox®, Allergan, Irvine, CA, USA) was reconstituted using non-preserved sterile saline solution 0.9%. Doses of BoNT-A were based on a previous report [20,29]. Bilateral intramuscular injections were performed in the masseter and anterior temporalis muscles using a 1-mL syringe with a 30-gauge needle by an investigator who was not involved in the dilution process. Subjects were asked to first clench their teeth to delimit the muscle area (masseter and anterior temporalis) and then relax the muscle whereafter a total of five injections per muscle with a separation of 5 mm between them were applied. Injections of BoNT-A or SS were performed during a single appointment. Participants and investigators assessing the outcomes were masked to all treatment assignments.

5.4. RDC/TMD Axis I Assessment

Mandibular movements and muscle sensitivity to palpation were evaluated in accordance with RDC/TMD-Axis I [3]. The RDC/TMD Axis I includes a clinical examination of range of mandibular movements and pain upon movement, assessment of joint sounds, and temporomandibular joint and muscle palpation. A diagnosis of MPF is based on pain-free opening capacity (mm) and number of muscle sites painful to palpation. Participants were evaluated while seated in a dental chair, in a room with adequate lighting. Clinical measurements of the mandibular movements were made by using a digital caliper rule (Mitutoyo 500- 144B—Suzano, São Paulo, Brazil), and included: pain-free opening, maximum unassisted and assisted opening, and right and left lateral movements. Palpation tests were performed bilaterally to six different areas of the face and head (origin, body, and insertion of masseter muscle and posterior, middle, and anterior temporalis muscle; the arithmetic mean of the three evaluation points in each muscle was considered for statistical analysis). Subjects' pain while palpation was recorded on a 4-point ordinal scale: 0 = no pain, 1 = mild pain, 2 = moderate pain, and 3 = severe pain.

5.5. Data Evaluation and Statistical Analyses

Data from mandibular movements and muscle tenderness to palpation were assessed at three time points: before, and 28 as well as 180 days after treatment. All variables' results were expressed as median, minimum, maximum, and means ± standard deviation (SD) and were assessed for normal distribution with the Shapiro–Wilk test. There was no normal distribution. Then, for non-parametric multiple comparison between groups Mann–Whitney U-test with Bonferroni correction was used. All data were analyzed using SPSS Statistics 25.0 software (IBM®, New York, NY, USA). A 5% probability level was considered significant in all tests.

Author Contributions: Conceptualization, G.D.l.T.C., M.E., A.C.M., L.R.B., B.R.D.S., A.M.A., R.L.P. and C.M.R.-B.; data curation, G.D.l.T.C., N.A.P. and R.L.P.; formal analysis, G.D.l.T.C., N.A.P., R.L.P., B.R.D.S. and A.M.A.; funding acquisition, G.D.l.T.C. and C.M.R.-B.; investigation, G.D.l.T.C., N.A.P. and R.L.P.; methodology, G.D.l.T.C., R.L.P., B.R.D.S., A.M.A., M.E., A.C.M., L.R.B. and C.M.R.-B.; project administration, G.D.l.T.C., M.E., A.C.M., L.R.B. and C.M.R.-B.; writing—original draft, G.D.l.T.C., R.L.P., N.A.P., B.R.D.S. and A.M.A.; writing—review and editing, G.D.l.T.C., R.L.P., B.R.D.S., A.M.A., A.C.M., M.E., L.R.B. and C.M.R.-B. All authors have read and agreed to the published version of the manuscript.

Funding: This study was financed by the Sao Paulo Research Foundation (FAPESP)—Brazil (grant number 2014/15863-7) and by national funds through the FCT—Foundation for Science and Technology, I.P., under the project UIDB/04585/2020.

Institutional Review Board Statement: The study was conducted according to the guidelines of the Declaration of Helsinki and approved by the Ethics Committee of Piracicaba Dental School—University of Campinas (CAAE # 22953113.8.0000.5418—Date: 4 February 2014).

Informed Consent Statement: Informed consent was obtained from all subjects involved in the study.

Acknowledgments: We acknowledge the Coordenação de Aperfeiçoamento de Pessoal de Nível Superior—Brasil (CAPES) Finance Code 001 for the Ph.D. scholarship of R. Lorenzi Poluha, and the Sao Paulo Research Foundation (FAPESP)—Brazil for the Post-Doctoral scholarship of G. De la Torre Canales (process 2017/21674-0) and the FCT—Foundation for Science and Technology, I.P., under the project (UIDB/04585/2020).

Conflicts of Interest: The funding sources were not involved in study design, collection, analysis and interpretation of data, decision to publish, or preparation of the manuscript. The authors declare no conflict of interest.

References

1. Manfredini, D.; Perinetti, G.; Guarda-Nardini, L. Dental malocclusion is not related to temporomandibular joint clicking: A logistic regression analysis in a patient population. *Angle Orthod.* **2014**, *84*, 310–315. [CrossRef] [PubMed]
2. Manfredini, D.; Ahlberg, J.; Winocur, E.; Guarda-Nardini, L.; Lobbezoo, F. Correlation of RDC/TMD axis I diagnoses and axis II pain-related disability. A multicenter study. *Clin. Oral. Investig.* **2011**, *15*, 749–756. [CrossRef] [PubMed]
3. Dworkin, S.F.; LeResche, L. Research diagnostic criteria for temporomandibular disorders: Review, criteria, examinations and specifications, critique. *J. Craniomandib. Disord.* **1992**, *6*, 301–355. [PubMed]
4. Schiffman, E.; Ohrbach, R.; Truelove, E.; Look, J.; Anderson, G.; Goulet, J.P.; List, T.; Svensson, P.; Gonzalez, Y.; Lobbezoo, F.; et al. Diagnostic Criteria for Temporomandibular Disorders (DC/TMD) for Clinical and Research Applications: Recommendations of the International RDC/TMD Consortium Network* and Orofacial Pain Special Interest Group. *J. Oral Facial Pain Headache* **2014**, *28*, 6–27. [CrossRef]
5. De la Torre Canales, G.; Bonjardim, L.R.; Poluha, R.L.; Carvalho Soares, F.F.; Guarda-Nardini, L.; Conti, P.R.; Manfredini, D. Correlation between Physical and Psychosocial Findings in a Population of Temporomandibular Disorder Patients. *Int. J. Prosthodont* **2020**, *33*, 155–159. [CrossRef] [PubMed]
6. Manfredini, D.; Favero, L.; Gregorini, G.; Cocilovo, F.; Guarda-Nardini, L. Natural course of temporomandibular disorders with low pain-related impairment: A 2-to-3-year follow-up study. *J. Oral Rehabil.* **2013**, *40*, 436–442. [CrossRef]
7. Greene, C.S. The etiology of temporomandibular disorders: Implications for treatment. *J. Orofac. Pain* **2001**, *15*, 93–105; discussion 106–116.
8. Guarda-Nardini, L.; Manfredini, D.; Salamone, M.; Salmaso, L.; Tonello, S.; Ferronato, G. Efficacy of botulinum toxin in treating myofascial pain in bruxers: A controlled placebo pilot study. *Cranio* **2008**, *26*, 126–135. [CrossRef]
9. Ferrillo, M.; Ammendolia, A.; Paduano, S.; Calafiore, D.; Marotta, N.; Migliario, M.; Fortunato, L.; Giudice, A.; Michelotti, A.; de Sire, A. Efficacy of rehabilitation on reducing pain in muscle-related temporomandibular dis-orders: A systematic review and meta-analysis of randomized controlled trials. *J. Back Musculoskelet. Rehabil.* **2022**. [CrossRef]
10. Deregibus, A.; Ferrillo, M.; Grazia Piancino, M.; Chiara Domini, M.; de Sire, A.; Castroflorio, T. Are occlusal splints effective in reducing myofascial pain in patients with muscle-related temporomandibular disorders? A randomized-controlled trial. *Turk. J. Phys. Med. Rehabil.* **2021**, *67*, 32–40. [CrossRef]
11. Kalladka, M.; Young, A.; Khan, J. Myofascial pain in temporomandibular disorders: Updates on etiopathogenesis and management. *J. Bodyw. Mov. Ther.* **2021**, *28*, 104–113. [CrossRef] [PubMed]
12. Deer, T.R.; Caraway, D.L.; Wallace, M.S. A definition of refractory pain to help determine suitability for device implantation. *Neuromodulation* **2014**, *17*, 711–715. [CrossRef] [PubMed]
13. Matak, I.; Bolcskei, K.; Bach-Rojecky, L.; Helyes, Z. Mechanisms of Botulinum Toxin Type A Action on Pain. *Toxins* **2019**, *11*, 459. [CrossRef] [PubMed]

14. Matak, I.; Lackovic, Z. Botulinum toxin A, brain and pain. *Prog. Neurobiol.* **2014**, *119–120*, 39–59. [CrossRef] [PubMed]
15. Munoz Lora, V.R.M.; Del Bel Cury, A.A.; Jabbari, B.; Lackovic, Z. Botulinum Toxin Type A in Dental Medicine. *J. Dent. Res.* **2019**, *98*, 1450–1457. [CrossRef] [PubMed]
16. Delcanho, R.; Val, M.; Nardini, L.G.; Manfredini, D. Botulinum Toxin for Treating Temporomandibular Disorders: What is the Evidence? *J. Oral Facial Pain Headache* **2022**, *36*, 6–20. [CrossRef]
17. Owen, M.; Gray, B.; Hack, N.; Perez, L.; Allard, R.J.; Hawkins, J.M. Impact of botulinum toxin injection into the masticatory muscles on mandibular bone: A systematic review. *J. Oral Rehabil.* **2022**, *49*, 644–653. [CrossRef]
18. Montes-Carmona, J.F.; Gonzalez-Perez, L.M.; Infante-Cossio, P. Treatment of Localized and Referred Masticatory Myofascial Pain with Botulinum Toxin Injection. *Toxins* **2020**, *13*, 6. [CrossRef]
19. Ernberg, M.; Hedenberg-Magnusson, B.; List, T.; Svensson, P. Efficacy of botulinum toxin type A for treatment of persistent myofascial TMD pain: A randomized, controlled, double-blind multicenter study. *Pain* **2011**, *152*, 1988–1996. [CrossRef]
20. de-la-Hoz, J.L.; de-Pedro, M.; Martin-Fontelles, I.; Mesa-Jimenez, J.; Chivato, T.; Bagues, A. Efficacy of botulinum toxin type A in the management of masticatory myofascial pain: A retrospective clinical study. *J. Am. Dent. Assoc.* **2022**, *153*, 683–691. [CrossRef]
21. Patel, A.A.; Lerner, M.Z.; Blitzer, A. IncobotulinumtoxinA Injection for Temporomandibular Joint Disorder. *Ann. Otol. Rhinol. Laryngol.* **2017**, *126*, 328–333. [CrossRef] [PubMed]
22. Cartagena-Sevilla, J.; Garcia-Fernandez, M.R.; Vicente-Villena, J.P. Analgesic Effect of Botulinum Toxin A in Myofascial Pain Syndrome Patients Previously Treated with Local Infiltration of Anesthetic and Steroids. *J. Pain Palliat. Care Pharm.* **2016**, *30*, 269–275. [CrossRef] [PubMed]
23. Kurtoglu, C.; Gur, O.H.; Kurkcu, M.; Sertdemir, Y.; Guler-Uysal, F.; Uysal, H. Effect of botulinum toxin-A in myofascial pain patients with or without functional disc displacement. *J. Oral Maxillofac. Surg.* **2008**, *66*, 1644–1651. [CrossRef] [PubMed]
24. Dressler, D.; Saberi, F.A.; Barbosa, E.R. Botulinum toxin: Mechanisms of action. *Arq. Neuropsiquiatr.* **2005**, *63*, 180–185. [CrossRef] [PubMed]
25. Cho, G.H.; Lee, Y. Analysis of Masticatory Muscle Activity Based on Presence of Temporomandibular Joint Disorders. *Med. Sci. Monit.* **2020**, *26*, e921337. [CrossRef]
26. Haggman-Henrikson, B.; Jawad, N.; Acuna, X.M.; Visscher, C.M.; Schiffman, E.; List, T. Fear of Movement and Catastrophizing in Participants with Temporomandibular Disorders. *J. Oral Facial Pain Headache* **2022**, *36*, 59–66. [CrossRef]
27. Merkle, S.L.; Sluka, K.A.; Frey-Law, L.A. The interaction between pain and movement. *J. Hand Ther.* **2020**, *33*, 60–66. [CrossRef]
28. Cote, J.N.; Hoeger Bement, M.K. Update on the relation between pain and movement: Consequences for clinical practice. *Clin. J. Pain* **2010**, *26*, 754–762. [CrossRef]
29. Favre-Guilmard, C.; Chabrier, P.E.; Kalinichev, M. Bilateral analgesic effects of abobotulinumtoxinA (Dysport((R))) following unilateral administration in the rat. *Eur. J. Pain* **2017**, *21*, 927–937. [CrossRef]
30. Pavone, F.; Luvisetto, S. Botulinum neurotoxin for pain management: Insights from animal models. *Toxins* **2010**, *2*, 2890–2913. [CrossRef]
31. De la Torre Canales, G.; Poluha, R.L.; Lora, V.M.; Araujo Oliveira Ferreira, D.M.; Stuginski-Barbosa, J.; Bonjardim, L.R.; Cury, A.; Conti, P.C.R. Botulinum toxin type A applications for masticatory myofascial pain and trigeminal neuralgia: What is the evidence regarding adverse effects? *Clin. Oral Investig.* **2019**, *23*, 3411–3421. [CrossRef] [PubMed]
32. De la Torre Canales, G.; Alvarez-Pinzon, N.; Munoz-Lora, V.R.M.; Vieira Peroni, L.; Farias Gomes, A.; Sanchez-Ayala, A.; Haiter-Neto, F.; Manfredini, D.; Rizzatti-Barbosa, C.M. Efficacy and Safety of Botulinum Toxin Type A on Persistent Myofascial Pain: A Randomized Clinical Trial. *Toxins* **2020**, *12*, 395. [CrossRef] [PubMed]

toxins

MDPI

Review

Cosmetic Treatment Using Botulinum Toxin in the Oral and Maxillofacial Area: A Narrative Review of Esthetic Techniques

Sung Ok Hong

Department of Oral and Maxillofacial Surgery, Kyung Hee University College of Dentistry, Kyung Hee University Hospital at Gangdong, Seoul 05278, Republic of Korea; catherine.so.hong.sleepdoc@gmail.com; Tel.: +82-02-440-7517

Abstract: Botulinum toxin (BoNT) is an anaerobic rod-shaped-neurotoxin produced by Clostridium botulinum, that has both therapeutic and lethal applications. BoNT injection is the most popular cosmetic procedure worldwide with various applications. Patients with dynamic wrinkles in areas such as the glabella, forehead, peri-orbital lines, nasal rhytides, and perioral rhytides are indicated. Excessive contraction of muscles or hyperactivity of specific muscles such as bulky masseters, cobble stone chins, gummy smiles, asymmetric smiles, and depressed mouth corners can achieve esthetic results by targeting the precise muscles. Patients with hypertrophic submandibular glands and parotid glands can also benefit esthetically. There are several FDA-approved BoNTs (obabotulinumtoxinA, abobotulinumtoxinA, incobotulinumtoxinA, letibotulinumtoxinA, prabotulinumtox-inA, daxibotulinumtoxinA, rimbotulinumtoxinB) and novel BoNTs on the market. This paper is a narrative review of the consensus statements of expert practitioners and various literature on the injection points and techniques, highlighting both the Asian and Caucasian population separately. This paper can serve as a practical illustrative guide and reference for optimal, safe injection areas and effective doses for application of BoNT in the face and oral and maxillofacial area. The history of BoNT indications, contraindications, and complications, and the merits of ultrasonography (US)-assisted injections are also discussed.

Keywords: botulinum toxin; Botox; cosmetic treatment; esthetic treatment; maxillofacial; dentist; injection; BoNT; non-invasive; face; wrinkles; aging; beauty; facial anatomy; toxin; rhytides

Key Contribution: This review focuses on esthetic procedures that both dentists and physicians can perform in the oral and maxillofacial areas. The injection amount of BoNT, depth, and points of forehead rhytides, glabella, crow's feet, infraorbital rhytides, bunny lines, perioral rhytides, bulky jaw, marionette lines, cobblestone chin, and gummy smile are discussed and animated in details based on expert panel opinion summaries.

Citation: Hong, S.O. Cosmetic Treatment Using Botulinum Toxin in the Oral and Maxillofacial Area: A Narrative Review of Esthetic Techniques. *Toxins* **2023**, *15*, 82. https://doi.org/10.3390/toxins15020082

Received: 30 November 2022
Revised: 13 January 2023
Accepted: 15 January 2023
Published: 17 January 2023

1. Introduction

Facial beauty, though slightly different in each ethnicity, tends to have a universal rule. A balanced, symmetrical, oval face with harmonious features is perceived as attractive and youthful [1–3]. Esthetic concerns are different by age groups with younger groups focusing more on a smooth contour and volume reduction, while older groups focus on wrinkles and improving volume loss [3]. Facial expression muscles are different from other muscular parts of the body because they have soft tissue attachments to the skin through the superficial musculoaponeurotic system, rather than to the bone [4]. Since contracting superficial skin moves in coordination with the underlying muscles, dynamic wrinkles perpendicular to the muscles develop [4,5]. These developed dynamic rhytides lead to atrophy of the dermis and pleating in the skin, which may give an impression of an angry, sad, or aging face. Botulinum neurotoxin (BoNT) can significantly soften dynamic wrinkles and even provide a lifting effect [6,7]. BoNT injection is the most popular cosmetic procedure worldwide with various applications. It can treat not only facial wrinkles but also a wide range of dermatologic, ophthalmologic, oral and maxillofacial, neurologic, urologic, and gynecologic conditions [8–11]. The reversible characteristics and versatile applications of BoNT make it widely preferable for both cosmetic and therapeutic treatment.

BoNT is a neurotoxin produced by the anaerobic rod-shaped bacterium *Clostridium botulinum*, and has both medical and lethal applications [12]. It is the most potent biological toxin known with an estimated lethal dose at 0.09 to 0.15 μg (IV or IM), 0.70 to 0.90 μg (inhalation), and 70 μg (PO) [11,13]. *C. botulinum* produces seven BoNT serotypes (A, B, C, D, E, F, G) [14,15]. An eighth serotype (X) was identified from *C. botulinum* strain 111 using bioinformatics techniques [15,16]. The most potent serotype is A, followed by B and F [17,18]. BoNT serotypes A and B are the only ones that have been manufactured for clinical use [7]. The effects of BoNT appear after approximately 2–3 days on rhytides and 3 weeks on larger muscles, and last between 3 and 6 months [19–21].

In 1829, a German medical officer and poet named Justinus Kerner (1786–1862) reported lethal food poisoning due to rotten sausages (*botulus*, Latin for sausage). In 1897, Emile von Ermengem investigated an outbreak of botulism due to raw ham in Belgium and found spore-forming anaerobic bacteria, *Bacillus botulinum* [19]. The outbreak of World War I and II weaponized BoNT by investigating the effect on muscle contraction [22]. In 1944, Edward Schantz cultured and isolated *C. botulinum*, and later in 1949, Arnold Burgen discovered the mechanism of how BoNT works by blocking acetylcholine release from the neuromuscular junction leading to muscular paralysis [11,23].

The first suggestion of using BoNT for therapeutic use was in 1973. An American ophthalmologist Alan B. Scott published the results of strabismus treatment using BoNT on monkeys. In 1977, he became the first person to use BoNT to treat blepharospasm and strabismus, and later founded the company Oculinum [24]. In 1987, Carruthers and Carruthers observed that BoNT treatment in patients with blepharospasm enhanced their glabellar lines and reported its cosmetic effect [25]. Soon after the United States Food and Drug Administration (FDA) approved BoNT in 1989, Oculinum was bought by Allergan in 1991, and Botox® was manufactured. After this, the FDA has approved BoNT for various cosmetic and non-cosmetic applications. Cosmetic applications for glabellar lines in 2002, severe axillary hyperhidrosis in 2004, migraines in 2010, lateral canthal lines in 2013, forehead lines in 2017 and sialorrhea in 2018 [9,26].The purpose of this review is to present an overview of BoNT and demonstrate the optimal, safe injection areas and effective dose for application of BoNT in the oral and maxillofacial area. This practical guideline depicts the anatomy of the facial muscles relative to the BoNT injection points and includes a narrative literature review.

2. Materials and Methods

This review explores quantitative data using a systematic search on studies depicting dose range and injection points from expert consensus opinions. A literature search was conducted using MEDLINE and PubMed electronic databases for the period from January 2002 to December 2022. Manual study searches were also performed using the reference list of articles included during the search process.

The inclusion criteria were as follows:

1. Studies in the English language;
2. Include dosage of BoNT and/or number of injection points;
3. Be performed in human adults with no diseases;
4. Given BoNT injection of the face for cosmetic or esthetic purpose;
5. The literature is limited to expert consensus.

Exclusion criteria were as follows:

1. Studies using BoNT for other reasons than cosmetic/aesthetic: i.e., stroke, neurogenic, bladder management, spasticity, sialorrhea, bruxism, strabismus, myofascial pain, TMJ, or obesity;

2. Studies using BoNT for cosmetic/aesthetic reasons in other parts of the body or other reasons: i.e., skin texture, scar, androgenic alopecia, neck wrinkles, trapezius hypertrophy, or calf hypertrophy;
3. Studies that investigated only a single muscle.

The search included the following keywords used in different combinations: "botox", "botulinum toxin", "consensus", "aesthetic", "cosmetic", "systematic review", and "face". The term "botox consensus" retrieved 202 studies, "botulinum toxin" AND "consensus" retrieved 315 studies. The search term "face botulinum toxin consensus" resulted in 56 studies, "esthetic botulinum toxin" AND "consensus" resulted in 54 articles, and "cosmetic botulinum toxin consensus" resulted in 42 studies. The term "botox systematic review" retrieved 421 articles.

3. Results

Titles and abstracts were screened, the eligibility criteria were applied, and full text analysis was performed in relevant publications. Thirty-three full text articles were screened for eligibility, of which six were excluded because of a lack of BoNT dosages and type of paper. A total of 27 articles were included in the literature review. The injection dosage and points proposed in this paper are based on the findings from such various reviews.

The BoNT dose and injection points from the views of expert opinions are summarized in Tables 1–3. A total of 27 consensus articles were reviewed after retrieving the data through a systematic search. Of the 27 studies, 4 were specified towards Asians, and therefore organized into a separate table (Table 3) [27–30]. Of the 23 other studies, those by Fagien et al. [31] and by Bertossi et al. [32] were each separately updated by the same group and therefore were excluded from the summary. Carruthers et al. [33] updated their consensus in 2008 and again in 2013 [34,35]. The initial 2004 consensus was grouped with the 2008 consensus, but the 2013 consensus was summarized because of slightly different parameters. Studies by Raspaldo et al. [36] and Gassia et al. [37] were identical to the 2010 consensus from Raspaldo et al. [38,39] and excluded from the summary tables. Most of the studies used onabotulinumtoxinA units, but three studies using different units of abobotulinumtoxinA were excluded from the review [40–42]. Three other studies using different BoNTA were included. Studies by Sundaram et al. [28] and Yutskovskay et al. [43] used incobotulinumtoxinA, while Ahn et al. [27] utilized Medytox. A total of 16 consensus papers were summarized in this narrative review (Tables 1–3).

Table 1. Consensus recommendations using Botulinum toxin A for the cosmetic treatment of various indications in the upper face.

Authors	Indication									
	Forehead		Glabella		Crow's Feet		Infraorbital		Bunny Lines	
	Total Dose (U) Dose per IP (U)	IP (n)	Total Dose (U) Dose per IP (U)	IP (n)	Total Dose (U) Dose per IP (U)	IP (n)	Total Dose (U) Dose per IP (U)	IP (n)	Total Dose (U) Dose per IP (U)	IP (n)
Carruthers et al., 2004, 2008 [33,34]	F: 6–15 M: 6–15	4–8	F: 10–30 M: 20–40	5–7	F: 10–30 M: 20–30	2–5/side	NR	NR	2–5	1/side
Carruthers et al., 2013 [35]	5–15	4–10	F: 10–50 M: 20–60	5–7	10–30	2–5/side	NR	NR	NR	NR
Raspaldo et al., 2011 [38,39]	F: 10–20 M: 10–30 1–2	3–5	8–25 4–5	2–5	6–16/side 2–4	3–4/side	2–4 0.5–2	1–2/side	4–8 2–4	1/side
Maas et al., 2012 [44]	11.75 (range: 5–30)	6	20 (range: 12–25)	5	20 (range: 6–30)	3/side	4 (range: 1.5–8)	1/side	6 (range: 2–12)	1/side
Imhof et al., 2013 [45]	F: 8 M: 12 0.5–2	4–6	20 4	5	4–6 1–3	3/side	2 0.5	2/side	2 1	1/side
Lorenc et al., 2013 [46]	F: 10–20 M: 20–40	4–6	20 (range: 10–40)	5	8–16/side	4/side	1 (range: 0.5–2.5)	1/side	NR	NR
Yuskovskaya et al., 2015 [43]	10–20 2–4	4–8	20 2–5	6	12/side 4	3/side	NR	NR	4–8 2–4	1/side
Sundaram et al., 2016 [47,48]	8–25 2–4	4–8	12–40 2–4	3–7	6–15/side 1–4	1–5/side	0.5–2/side 0.5–2	1–3/side	4–8,10 2–4	2–3
De Maio et al., 2017 [49–51]	NR	5–7	NR	5	NR	3/side	NR	1/side	4–6 2	2 or 3
Kaminer et al., 2020 [52]	F: 2–20 M: 4–30	2–12	F: 6–35 M: 8–40	3–8	6–20	2–6/side	NR	NR	2–10	1–2/side
Signorini et al., 2022 [53]	20 2–4	5–10	30 6	5–7	18 6	3/side	1–2 0.5–1	1/side	4–6 2–3	1/side

U, unit; IP, injection point; n, number; F, female; M, male; NR, not reported; Up, upper lip; L, lower lip.

Table 2. Consensus recommendations for patients using BoNT for the cosmetic treatment of various indications in the lower face.

Authors	Indication											
	Perioral		Gummy Smile		Masseter Hypertrophy		Parotid Gland Hypertrophy		DAO		Cobble Stone Chin	
	Total Dose (U) Dose per IP (U)	IP (n)	Total Dose (U) Dose per IP (U)	IP (n)	Total Dose (U) Dose per IP (U)	IP (n)	Total Dose (U) Dose per IP (U)	IP (n)	Total Dose (U) Dose per IP (U)	IP (n)	Total Dose (U) Dose per IP (U)	IP (n)
Carruthers et al., 2004, 2008 [33,34]	4–5	2–6	2–4	1/side	25–30/side	NR	NR	NR	2–5	1/side	4–5	1–2
Carruthers et al., 2013 [35]	4–6	2–6	NR	NR	NR	NR	NR	NR	1–15 1–7.5	1/side	4–10	1–2
Raspaldo et al., 2011 [38,39]	Up: 2–5 L: 2–5 ~1	Up: 2–4 L: 2–4	3–5/side 1–2	1/side	18–30/side 6	1–5/side	NR	NR	2–5/side 1–2.5	1–2/side	6–10 3–5	2
Maas et al., 2012 [44]	5 (range: 2–12)	Up: 4 L: 2	5 (range: 2–10)	1/side	32.5 (range: 20–60)	3/side	NR	NR	6 (range: 2–10)	1/side	5 (range: 3–10)	2–3
Imhof et al., 2013 [45]	4	Up: 4 L: 2	NR	NR	4–6 2	2 or 3	NR	NR	1–3	1/side	6 (range: 2–8)	2
Lorenc et al., 2013 [46]	5 2.5	2	NR	NR	NR	NR	NR	NR	5 2.5	1/side	4–5	2
Yuskovskaya et al., 2015 [43]	Up: 4–6 1–1.5	Up: 4	NR	NR	50 2	3/side	NR	NR	6 3	1/side	6 3	2
Sundaram et al., 2016 [47,48]	1–5 0.5–1	2–5	1–4, 8 0.5–2	1–2/side	15–40 5–15	1–5/side	NR	NR	2–4/side 2	1–2/side	4–10 2–3	1–4
De Maio et al., 2017 [49–51]	Up: 2–4 L: 2 1	U: 2–4 L: 2	6–10 2	3–5	6–24/side 4–8	3/side	NR	NR	4–8 2–4	1/side	4–8 2.5	1- 3
Kaminer et al., 2020 [52]	2–10	2–8	NR	NR	5–35	2–6/side	NR	NR	2–6	1–2/side	2–10	1–4
Signorini et al., 2022 [53]	1–4 0.5–1	Up: 2–4	6–10 2	3	25–50/side 5–10 or 7–22	3–5/side	NR	NR	4–8 2–4	1/side	8–10 4–10	1–2

U, unit; IP, injection point; n, number; F, female; M, male; NR, not reported; Up, upper lip; L, lower lip.

Table 3. Consensus recommendations for Asian patients using BoNT for the cosmetic treatment of various indications.

Indication	Authors											
	Ahn et al., 2013 [27]			Wu et al., 2016 [30]			Sundaram et al., 2016 [28]			Kapoor et al., 2017 [29]		
	Total Dose (U)	Dose per IP (U)	IP (n)	Total Dose (U)	Dose per IP (U)	IP (n)	Total Dose (U)	Dose per IP (U)	IP (n)	Total Dose (U)	Dose per IP (U)	IP (n)
Forehead rhytides	6–13.5	1–1.5	6–9	5–12	1–4	NR	12–14 (range: 2–32)	0.1–5	12	F: 6–8 M: 10–12	NR	4–6
Glabella	8	4	3	12–20	NR	3–10	10–20 (range: 6–25)	2–4	3–5	16–20	NR	5–7
Crow's feet	14	2–3	3/side	6–12/side	1–4	NR	6–9 (range: 4–16)/side	2–4	3–4/side	8–12/side	NR	3–4/side
Infraorbital rhytides	1–2	0.5	2–4	4–6	NR	NR	1–2	0.5–1	2–3/side	n/a	NR	NR
Bunny lines	6	2	3	4–6	NR	NR	3–4	0.5–5	2	2–4/side	1–2	2
Perioral rhytides	0.8–1.2	0.2–0.3	4	2–8	NR	NR	2–3 (range: 1–8)	0.5–1	2–6	2–4	NR	Up: 4 L: 2
Gummy smile	4–6	2–3	1/side	2–12	NR	NR	2–4	1–2	2	2–3/side	NR	2
Bulky jaw	24–30/side	8–10	3/side	40–80	NR	NR	20–40	4–6	3–5/side	15–30/side	NR	3/side
Parotid gland hypertrophy	NR	NR	NR	NR	NR	NR	20–40/side	4–6	4–6	NR	NR	NR
DAO	6–10	3–5	1/side	4–6	NR	NR	2–4/side	2–4	1/side	2–3/side	NR	1/side
Cobblestone chin	mild: 5 severe: 10	5	mild: 1 severe: 2	4–8	NR	NR	8 (range: 2–16)	2–4	1–2/side	6–8	NR	1–2

U, unit; IP, injection points; n, number; F, female; M, male; NR, not reported; Up, upper lip; L, lower lip.

3.1. *Cosmetic Indications and Contraindications*

Elucidating the cosmetic indications and contraindications of BoNT is crucial to maximize patient satisfaction and minimize complications. Patients with dynamic wrinkles, which are formed during facial expression are indicated [4]. Areas with dynamic motion such as the glabella, forehead, peri-orbital lines, nasal rhytides, and perioral rhytides are common injection areas [7,54,55]. Patients with static wrinkles that are present at rest can also be candidates. However, the results are less dramatic and additional treatment sessions or additional esthetic procedures, such as fillers, may be required to achieve ideal outcomes. Excessive contraction of muscles or hyperactivity of specific muscles can also cause non-cosmetic appearances. Patients with bulky masseters, cobble stone chins, gummy smiles, asymmetric smiles, depressed mouth corners, brow ptosis, flaring nostrils, depressed nasal tips, temporal hypertrophy, and trapezius hypertrophy can achieve esthetic results by targeting the precise muscles [7,22]. Patients with hypertrophic submandibular glands and parotid glands can also benefit esthetically in select cases [56].

Contraindications include immunocompromised patients with neuromuscular disorders, such as myasthenia gravis and Lambert–Eaton syndrome; neurodegenerative diseases such as amyotrophic lateral sclerosis; and pregnancy and breast-feeding [4,19]. BoNT is also contraindicated in patients with unrealistic expectations, body dysmorphic syndrome, keloidal scarring, active dermatoses or infection in the treatment area, motor weakness in the treatment area (Bell's palsy), and allergic reactions to BoNT constituents (cow's milk protein allergy using abobotulinumtoxinA) [57]. Theoretical drug interactions between BoNT and aminoglycoside antibiotics, quinidine, calcium channel blocker, magnesium sulfate, succihylcholine, and polymyxin exist [22,58,59].

3.2. Cosmetically Used Botulinum Toxin Products

Currently, there are several popular FDA-approved (six BoNTA, one BoNTB) and non-approved toxin products on the market (Table 4) [8,12,60,61]. BoNTs vary in composition, complex size, molecular and chemical properties, supply form, and immunogenicity. Pure BoNT is manufactured as 150 kDa proteins that bind in different quantities to neurotoxin-associated complexing proteins (NAPs) to form high-molecular-weight progenitor complexes [8,62]. Commercial BoNT products have different complements of NAPs, which lead to the formation of various molecular weights and three-dimensional structures [62]. Excipients are added to ensure long-term storage and minimize inactive neurotoxins because they might not interact with nerve cells but are recognized by the immune system [63].

Table 4. Summary of cosmetically used BoNT. The active substances, excipients, and stabilization form per vial, and the commercial brand names are shown.

US FDA-Approved Generic Name	Active Substance	Excipient	Unit/ Vial	Stabilization (form)	Commercial Products
OnabotulinumtoxinA	Complex (900 kDa)	HSA 0.5 mg, NaCl 0.9 mg	100	Vacuum-dried (P)	Botox®, Botox Cosmetic®, Vistabel®, Vistabex®
AbobotulinumtoxinA	Complex (500–900 kDa)	HSA 0.125 mg, Lactose 2.5 mg	500	Lyophilized (P)	Dysport®, Reloxin®, Azzalure®
IncobotulinumtoxinA	Complex-free (150 kDa)	HSA 1 mg, Sucrose 4.7 mg L-methionine (q.s.)	100	Lyophilized (P)	Xeomin® Bocouture®
LanbotulinumtoxinA	Complex (900 kDa)	Gelatin 5 mg, Dextran 25 mg, Sucrose 25 mg	100	Lyophilized (P)	BTXA®, Prosigne®, Lantox®
LetibotulinumtoxinA	Complex	HSA 0.5 mgNaCl 0.9 mg	100	Lyophilized (P)	Botulax®, Regenox®, Zentox®
PrabotulinumtoxinA	Complex (900 kDa)	HSA 0.5 mgNaCl 0.9 mg	100	Vacuum-dried (P)	Nabota®, Jeuveau®, Nuceiva®
N/A	Complex (940 kDa)	HSA 0.5 mgNaCl 0.9 mg	100	Lyophilized (P)	Meditoxin®, Neuronox®
N/A	Complex (900 kDa)	Gelatin 6 mg, Maltose 12 mg	100	Lyophilized (P)	Relatox®
N/A	Complex	Polysorbate	25	L	Innotox®
N/A	Complex-free (150 KDa)	Polysorbate 20 (q.s.) Sucrose 3 mg NaCl 0.9 mg	100	Lyophilized (P)	Coretox®
DaxibotulinumtoxinA	Purified toxin (150 kDa)	Peptide (RTP004) Polysorbate 20 sugar	100	Lyophilized (P)	DAXXIFY®
RimabotulinumtoxinB	Complex (700 kDa)	HSA 0.5 mg NaCl 5.844 mg Sodium succinate 1.621 mg	5000	L	Neurobloc®, Myobloc®

HSA, Human Serum Albumin; NACL, sodium chloride; P, powder; L, liquid; q.s., quantum sufficit.

3.3. Facial Target Muscles and Injection Doses

Accurately administered injections and detailed knowledge of the anatomy to determine the correct depth and injection points are important factors for minimizing complications. The relevant anatomy including the muscles involved and amount of injection, is shown in Table 5 [20,28,44,55,60]. Thorough comprehension of the facial musculature and adjacent anatomy is essential before treatment initiation. Diffusion of BoNT differs according to the amount of mixed saline. However, in general, 1–5 mL of saline is mixed with 100 U of BoNTA, which results in diffusion distances 2.5–3 cm in diameter [4,20,64]. Before injection, good lighting, marking injection points, prefilling syringes with the required dose, and pre-photography are beneficial.

Table 5. Facial treatment areas in correlation with the target muscles, total amount of botulinum toxin, and number of injection points.

Facial Treatment Areas	Target Muscles	Total Dose	Dose per IP	Number of IP
Forehead rhytides	Frontalis	6–20 U	0.5–1 U	4–6/row (2 rows)
Glabella (Frown lines)	Corrugator supercilia, Procerus, Depressor supercilii	12–30 U	2–4 U	3–5
Crow's feet (Lateral canthal lines)	Lateral orbicularis oculi	4–16 U/side	2–4 U	3–4/side
Infraorbital rhytides	Orbicularis oculi	2–4 U	0.5–1 U	2–3/side
Bunny lines (Nasal rhytides)	Nasalis (transverse) Levator labii superioris alaeque nasi	3–4 U	1.5–2 U	2
Perioral rhytides (lipstick lines, smoker's lines)	Orbicularis oris	2–3 U	0.5 U	4–6
Gummy smile	Levator labii superioris, Levator labii superioris alaeque nasi, Zygomaticus minor	2–6 U	1–2 U	1–2/side
Bulky jaw	Masseter	15–30 U/side	5 U	3–5/side
Hypertrophic parotid gland	Parotid gland	20–40 U	4–6 U	4–6/side
Drooping oral commissures (frown lines, DAO)	Depressor anguli oris	4–10 U	2–5 U	2
Cobblestone chin	Mentalis	8–10 U	2–4 U	2

U, unit; IP, insertion point. Numbers in the table are adapted from consensus literature summarized in Tables 1–3.

3.4. *Injection Techniques of BoNT in the Face*

BoNT injection depth and amounts differ within each area of the face. Intramuscular injections act on the neuromuscular end plate, leading to denervation of the muscles and subsequent relaxation [19]. Injections can be subdermal in areas where the muscles are very superficial, such as the orbicularis oculi and frontalis muscles. The maximum injection dosage should be injected into the muscle origin, where action is the strongest. Muscles with fibers inserted into the skin can be injected intradermally. Moreover, superficial fibers can be targeted subdermally [4].

3.4.1. Forehead Frontalis

Contraction of the frontalis muscle leads to wrinkles on the forehead. This muscle is the only elevator muscle of the upper face originating from the galeal aponeurotic and is inserted into the subcutaneous level and deep dermis of the skin on the superciliary arch. The forehead has high variability due to the diverse individualized animation patterns during facial expressions. The key is to leave the forehead with little activity without leaving a frozen look. Intracutaneous injection of 15–20 U should be targeted at least 1–2 cm above (higher in aged individuals) the orbital rim to prevent brow ptosis (Figure 1). Lateral injection points should extend 2 cm laterally from the eyebrow to minimize excessive lifting of the eyebrow that may lead to a "samurai" or "Spock" look [19,56]. The lateral border of the frontalis muscle is situated 1 cm lateral to the superior temporal crest, which is on the same perpendicular plane as the lateral eyebrow tail [65]. When the BoNT injection point is too medial, diffusion into the lateral portion of the frontalis muscle is difficult and may cause such a look.

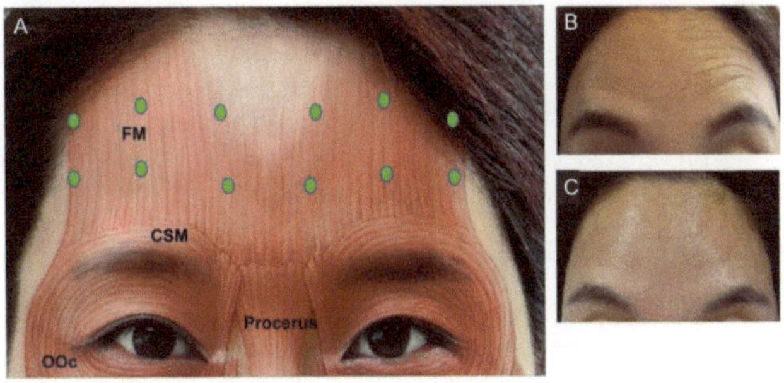

Figure 1. Frontalis muscles. (**A**) Injection points (green dot), facial photographs (**B**) before injection, (**C**) after injection. FM, frontalis muscle; OOc, orbicularis oculi; CSM, corrugator supercilia.

3.4.2. Glabella

Wrinkles in this area are formed by continuous action of the procerus and corrugator supercilii muscles, which are brow depressors. They are formed as a result of frowning and may exist as static vertical lines if left untreated in the dynamic state. The corrugator supercilii originates from the medial supraorbital ridge, thickening and thinning laterally [55]. The muscle lies below the frontalis muscle and injections should be intramuscular and deep. The procerus muscle originates from the periosteum of the nasal bone and upper lateral cartilages, and inserts into the glabellar skin and fibers of the frontalis muscle [56].

In total, 12 U to 20 U of BoNT should be injected into 3 to 5 points (Figure 2). Three injection points are usually required in Asian women. Additionally, five-point injections are helpful in men or patients with bulkier glabellas [28]. The injection point for the procerus muscle should be marked at the intersection of the two lines drawn from the medial brow to the contralateral medial canthus. Injection into the corrugator supercilia is deeper in the medial part and slightly superficial on the lateral side. To avoid brow ptosis, injections should not pass through the mid-pupillary line. Injections should be 1 cm superior to the upper inner boundary of the orbital rim to minimize blepharoptosis. This occurs when toxin spreads to the levator palpebrae superioris muscle, making apparent disfigurement and movement of the eyes difficult. The needle should also point upward at a 30° angle [56,66].

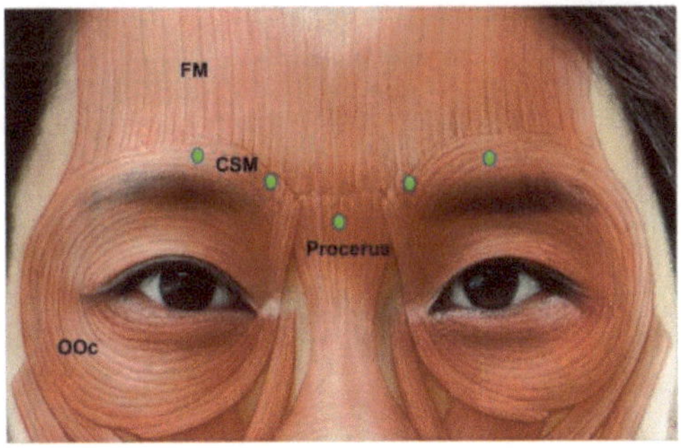

Figure 2. Glabella injection points. FM, frontalis muscle; OOc, orbicularis oculi; CSM, corrugator supercilia.

3.4.3. Lateral Canthal Lines (Crow's Feet)

Crow's feet are caused by contraction of the superficially situated orbicularis oculi muscle. It is a sphincter muscle encircling the orbit and is divided into three portions: palpebral, orbital, and lacrimal [33]. The muscle originates from the nasal part of the frontal bone, the medial palpebral ligament, and the frontal process of the maxilla. The most peripheral preorbital part causes protrusion of the eyebrow and voluntary eye closure is the target of BoNT [67]. Wrinkles in this area can be seen starting in patients aged approximately 20–25 years old [19]. To minimize complications, 6 U to 12 U of BoNT per side should be injected intracutaneously, producing a wheal (Figure 3). Three injections should be targeted 1.5 cm lateral to the lateral canthus or 1 cm outside the bony orbital wall to reduce the chances of diplopia, ectropion, and drooping of the lower eyelid [33]. To prevent asymmetrical smiles, injections should not be targeted close to the inferior margin of the zygoma. This area is susceptible to bruising due to the high vascularity [35,49].

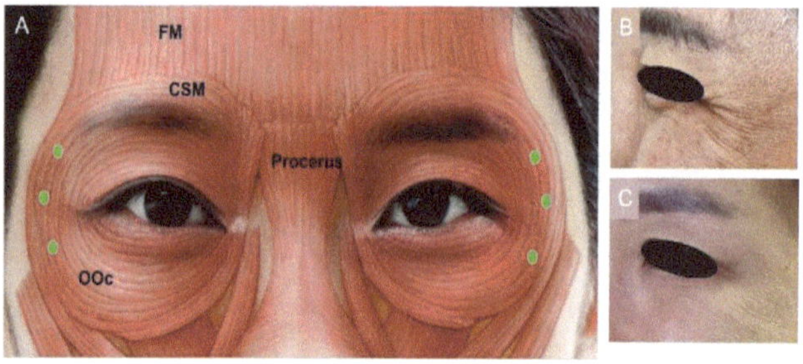

Figure 3. Lateral canthal (**A**) injection points, (**B**) before injection, (**C**) after injection. FM, frontalis muscle; OOc, orbicularis oculi; CSM, corrugator supercilia.

3.4.4. Infraorbital Rhytides

The palpebral part of the lower eyelid closes the eyelid and is subdivided into preseptal and pretarsal portions [49]. Subdermal injection of 2 U to 4 U of BoNT should be administered into the junction of the pretarsal and preseptal portions of the orbicularic oculi (Figure 4). To possess a "charming roll" in the pretarsal area, which makes the patient appear youthful, injections should be distanced from the lower ciliary margin [28]. Medial infraorbital BoNT injection doses should be minimal and injection delicate to prevent lower eyelid edema [28]. Patients with a positive snap test, lower eyelid puffiness, and previous lower lid blepharoplasty are not good candidates because scleral show may result in complications [49].

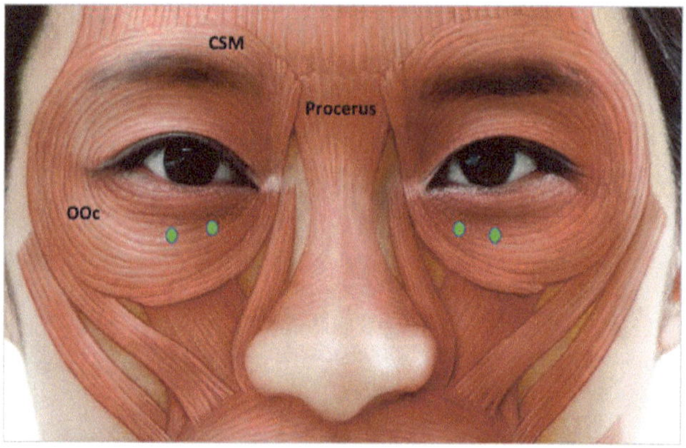

Figure 4. Infraorbital rhytides injection points. OOc, orbicularis oculi; CSM, corrugator supercilia.

3.4.5. Bunny Lines

Bunny lines are created by contraction of the transverse nasalis muscle, which draws the nose up and medially [50]. Other muscles such as the procerus, levator labii superioris alaeque nasi (LLSAN), and medial fibers of the orbicularis oculi may also have minor contributions. Intramuscular BoNT injections of 3 U to 4 U should be performed slightly lateral to the mid nose bridge (Figure 5). A third medial injection on the bridge of the nose can be performed in severe cases [50]. Injections that are too lateral or inferior may lead to lip drooping if BoNT is diffused into the levator labii superioris (LLS), levator anguli oris, or LLSAN muscles [67].

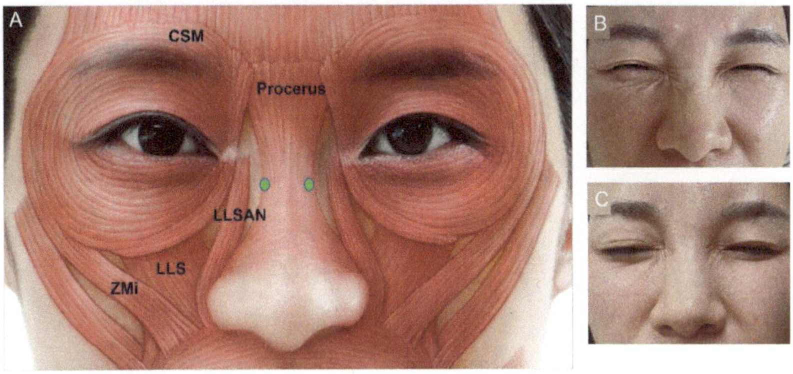

Figure 5. Bunny lines (**A**) injection points, (**B**) before injection, (**C**) after injection. LLSAN, levator labii superioris alaeque nasi; LLS, levator labii sup; Zmi, zygomaticus minor; CSM, corrugator supercilia.

3.4.6. Gummy Smile

A symmetrical smile with 1–2 mm gingival exposure is perceived as an esthetic smile [68,69]. Gummy smile is defined as an excessive gingival display greater than 3 mm when smiling. Mazzuco and Hexsel [70] further subclassified the gummy smile into four types: anterior, posterior, mixed, and asymmetric. In moderate gummy smile, the LLSAN elevates and everts the upper lip, while the depressor septi nasi muscle pulls the nasal tip down. In severe gummy smile, the LLS and to a lesser extent the zygomaticus minor (ZMi) also raise the upper lip. A single-point injection of 2 U on each side, 1 cm lateral to the nostril ala, also known as the Yonsei point, can target these three muscles (Figure 6) [56,71].

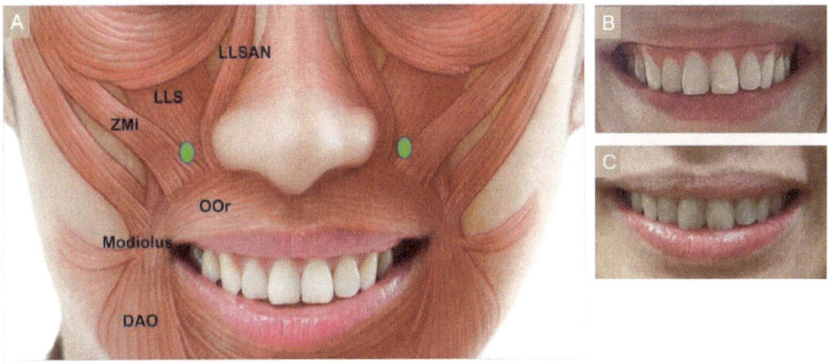

Figure 6. Gummy smile (**A**) injection points, (**B**) before injection, (**C**) after injection. LLSAN, Levator labii superioris alaeque nasi; LLS, Levator labii superioris; Zmi: zygomaticus minor; OOr: orbicularis oris, DAO: depressor anguli oris.

3.4.7. Perioral Rhytides

Dynamic vertical rhytides in this area are due to sphincter action of the orbicular oris muscle. The orbicularis oris originates from the modiolus, mandible, and the maxilla near the incisor fossa and inserts into the skin of lips encircling the upper and lower lips [67]. The treatment of vertical perioral wrinkles requires patient to contract the lips. Depending on anatomy, intracutaneous and intradermal injections can be administered. In total, 2–3 U of BoNT should be injected along the vermilion border (Figure 7). Flattening of the vermilion border can be a secondary complication due to contraction of the orbicularis oris. However, this can be easily corrected using dermal fillers. Since functional competency, facial asymmetry, lip depression, or lip elevation might occur, low doses of BoNT are recommended [44].

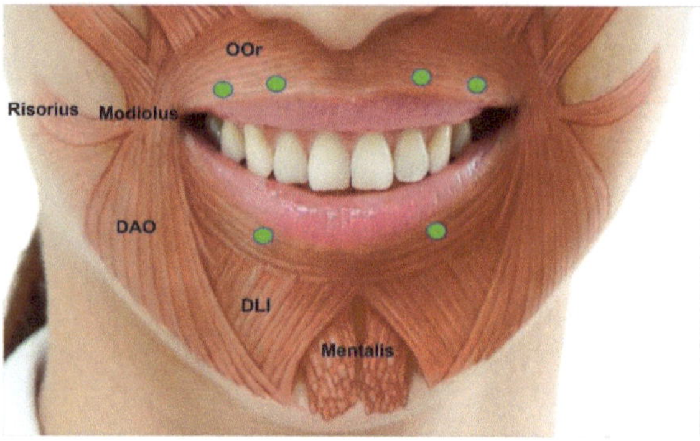

Figure 7. Perioral rhytides injection points. OOR, orbicularis oris; DAO, depressor anguli oris; DLI, depressor labii inferioris.

3.4.8. Masseter Hypertrophy

The masseter muscle is one of the four masticatory muscles that facilitates chewing and causes mouth closing. It is a superficial quadrangular muscle that originates from the zygomatic arch and attaches to the lateral border and the angle of the mandible [56]. Particularly in Asian women, a small oval face with a non-square angle and smooth jaw contour is perceived as esthetically appealing. Since hypertrophy of the masseter leads to a broad face, reduction in the muscle using BoNT has become a popular procedure in Asian countries.

Injections need to be both deep and superficial to effectively reduce the large muscle because a deep inferior tendon (DIT) can block diffusion into both levels, causing paradoxical masseteric bulging [65]. Typically, 25 U to 30 U of BoNT can be injected on each side of the masseter (Figure 8). Injection points can be modified in smaller muscles and skinnier patients to minimize diffusion of the toxin anteriorly, which may leave a "sunken cheek" appearance. Injection too anterior or superiorly can also cause "sunken cheek". Deeply injecting below a line drawn from the mouth corner to the tragus and at least 1 cm away from the anterior border of the masseter muscle is advisable [72,73]. Injection into the masseter can also reduce bruxism, clenching, and myofascial pain symptoms. However excessive doses of BoNT may temporarily cause difficulty in chewing.

3.4.9. Parotid Gland Hypertrophy

The parotid gland is an inverted-pyramidal-shaped organ that lies on the posterior border of the mandible angle [56,74]. Due to congenital, iatrogenic, or acquired conditions, BoNT in the glands plays a role in the esthetically slimming volume of the hypertrophic glands. BoNT can block not only the acetylcholine from binding in the neuromuscular junction but also in the salivary gland [28,75]. Initially, BoNT was used to treat sialorrhea. However, injection to reduce benign hypertrophy of the salivary glands has also been reported [65]. When the mandibular contour is bulky and extends below the angle, parotid gland hypertrophy could be suspected. Since the parotid gland lies superficial to the masseter muscle, 20 U to 30 U of BoNT should be injected more superficially than the masseter (Figure 9) [28]. Since the majority of salivary production comes from the submandibular gland, high-dose injections simultaneously into both the parotid gland and submandibular gland in patients may lead to severe dry mouth [56,76,77].

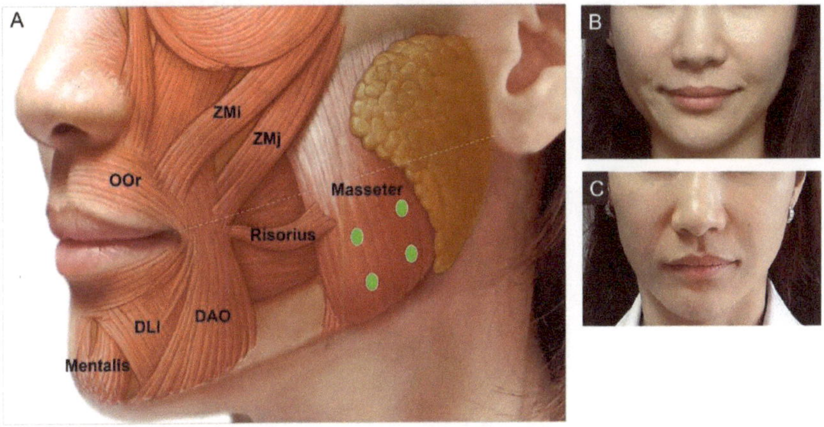

Figure 8. Masseter (**A**) injection points, (**B**) before injection, (**C**) after injection. Zmi, zygomaticus minor; ZMj, zygomaticus major; OOr, orbicularis oris; DAO, depressor anguli oris; DLI, depressor labii inferioris.

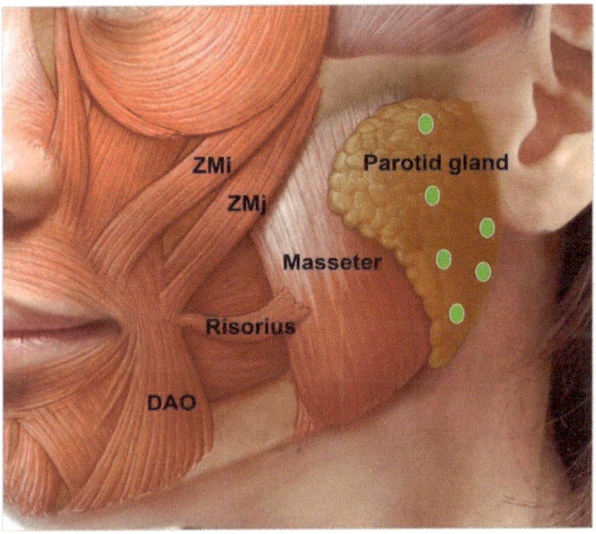

Figure 9. Parotid gland injection points. Zmi, zygomaticus minor; ZMj, zygomaticus major; DAO, depressor anguli oris.

3.4.10. Drooping Oral Commissures

The depressor anguli oris (DAO) muscle originates from the oblique line of the mandible and inserts into the modiolus [4,66]. Excessive contraction of the depressor anguli oris muscle pulls the mouth corners down creating a drooping and sad impression. Subdermally or intradermally 4 U to 10 U of BoNT can be injected, 1 cm lateral and lower to the mouth corner (Figure 10) [51]. In Asian patients, since the modiolus is situated in a lower position than in Caucasians, injection can be even lower [56]. Injection into the depressor labii inferior could cause difficulty in sipping water, while imprecise targeting of the muscles can lead to an asymmetrical smile.

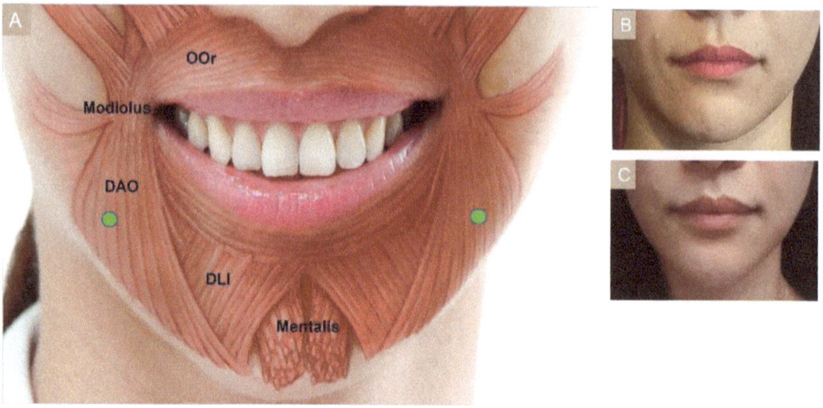

Figure 10. Depressor anguli oris (DAO) (**A**) injection points, (**B**) before injection, (**C**) after injection. OOr, orbicularis oris; DAO, depressor anguli oris; DLI, depressor labii inferioris.

3.4.11. Cobble Stone Chin

The mentalis muscle is a lower lip levator, which changes the chin texture when hyperactivated. This muscle originates from the alveolar bone inferior to the lateral incisor and attaches medially towards the skin, forming a dome-shaped chin [56]. A pebbled or dimpled appearance of the chin can be treated with two injections, totaling 10 U into the mentalis muscle (Figure 11). Injection too superiorly in proximity to the lower lip can spread BoNT to the orbicularis oris, and too laterally to the DAO. BoNT diffusion into both muscles may lead to ptosis or asymmetry of the lower lip [51]. It is important to remain at least 1 cm below the mental sulcus to avoid oral incompetence [55].

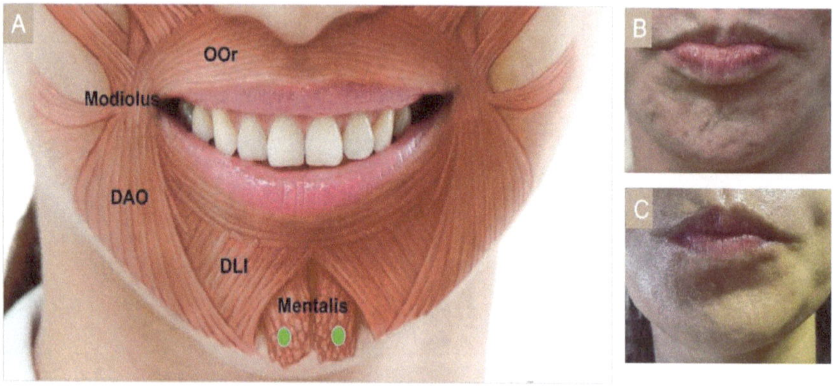

Figure 11. Mentalis (**A**) injection points, (**B**) before injection, (**C**) after injection. OOr, orbicularis oris; DAO, depressor anguli oris; DLI, depressor labii inferioris.

3.5. Ultrasonography (US)-Guided Botulinum Toxin Techniques

To maximize accuracy and minimize complications, US-guided treatments have been actively utilized in minimally invasive esthetic treatments, such as BoNT, fillers, and threads [65,78,79]. US is useful for distinguishing between anatomical structures such as vessels, muscle, fat, bone, and glands [66]. Not only can anatomical landmarks be seen in real time, but also injection needles and cannulas can be visualized during the procedures, which make outcomes more predictable (Figure 12). Therapy can be reproducible, which increases the efficacy and safety of esthetic treatments. Rather than injecting blindly into a muscle or layer, BoNT can accurately target a selected area and thereby treat the asymmetry in patients with crooked smiles or even deviated lower faces [80,81].

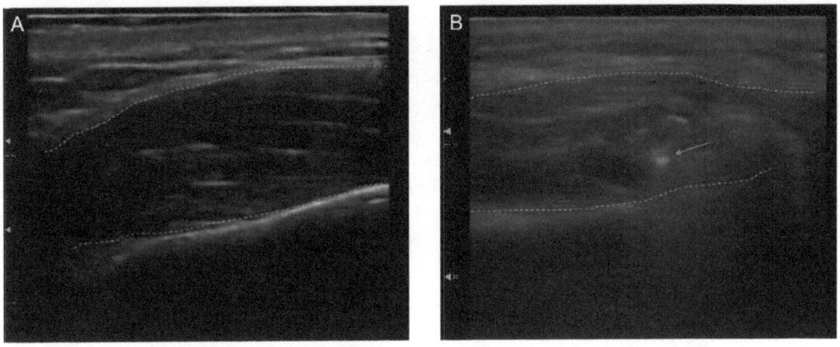

Figure 12. Ultrasonography imaging with outline of the muscle (yellow dotted line) (**A**) masseter, (**B**) masseter with needle tip (orange arrow).

3.6. Complications

BoNT is generally considered to have a wide safety margin in terms of risk. However, since its use has become more common, various injection-related adverse effects (AE) have arisen. Complications are usually technique-dependent, and their incidence decreases as the injector becomes experienced [57]. Complications are the result of reactions to the injection itself or due to the spread of BoNT to untargeted areas [57,82]. Injection-related reactions, such as erythema, edema, and injection pain, are usually mild and temporary and resolve within days. Bruising and ecchymosis are common but tend to take longer to resolve. A recent systematic review reported complication rates in the upper face to be 16% [83]. Headaches and migraines were the most frequently reported AE and this may be related to periosteal trauma or intramuscular hematoma formation during injection [83,84]. Anxiety, vasovagal episodes, paresthesia or dysesthesia, and allergic reactions should also be closely monitored [4,57]. Undesired effects due to the distant spread of BoNT include blepharoptosis, eyebrow ptosis, undesired eyebrow shape, unnatural face, eye opening difficulty, and unsatisfactory results [73,85]. Temporary blepharoptosis is seen in approximately 1–5% of patients [4]. Nasopharyngitis, sinusitis, blurred vision, upset stomach, voice changes, restricted mouth opening, muscle atrophy, and stiffness were also adverse events (AEs) encountered after injection [9,22,84].

The development of neutralizing antibodies is a crucial AE. BoNT may be regarded as a foreign substance in the body that induces an immune response after repeated treatment [86]. Therefore, to reduce antigen occurrence, a commercial product with a low risk of antigenicity should be selected, such as that with fewer complex proteins. Another way to minimize the risk of neutralizing antibody formation is to use the minimum dose needed for effect, injected at least 3 months apart, and avoid booster injections within one month [87,88].

4. Discussion

Several expert consensus statements have also been published from various parts of the world including Europe, Pan-Asia, and the Americas [28,33–35,38,44–53]. The results are shown in Tables 1–3 and in the supplementary table (Table S1). There are also numerous systematic reviews related to dosing and effective injections of BoNT. A Cochrane systematic review by Camargo et al. [54] in 2021 looked at 14,919 people (mostly women) from 65 RCTs to see if BoNTA was safe and effective in facial wrinkles. Different types of BoNT were compared with a placebo or each other in cases where glabellar lines, crow's feet, perioral lines, and forehead lines were treated. The study found that at 4 weeks after injection, all types of BoNT reduced glabellar lines more than the placebo. Regarding safety, ptosis was the only major AE reported and it was seen in fewer than 5% of the trials [54]. The dose range according to the facial region and BoNT brand was also investigated. The dose for glabella lines using onabotulinumtoxinA was 8 U to 80 U, abobotulinumtoxinA was 20 U to 75 U, incobotulinumtoxinA was 20 U to 24 U, daxibotulinumtoxinA was 20 U to 60 U, NewBoNTA (Medytox®, Prostigne®, Neuronox®) was 20 U, LiquidBoNTA was 20 U to 75 U, and prabotulinumtoxinA was 20 U to 60 U [89–91]. The dose for forehead lines using onabotulinumtoxinA was 10 U to 48 U, and incobotulinumtoxinA was 10 U to 20 U [92,93]. For crow's feet the dose using onabotulinumtoxinA was 7.5 U to 24 U, abobotulinumtoxinA was 30 U, incobotulinumtoxinA was 7.5 U to 12 U, and Neuronox® was 24 U [90,94]. Perioral lines were treated with 7.5 U to 12 U of onabotulinumtoxinA [95,96]. The distribution of injection points for the glabellar lines were three to seven points. It was four to eight for the forehead, three points for the crow's feet, and four points for the perioral lines. The dose and injection areas seem to differ for all types of BoNTAs for each area. Some BoNTA types have similar efficacy, but some areas require more Units for similar effect. Still, the data comparing different types of BoNT are limited, and with the evolution of newer BoNT brands, further investigation is needed to find the accurate efficacy and dose.

The injections points vary slightly between culture and ethnicity, and with sex. In general, men need greater amounts of BoNT injection because they tend to have thicker skin, more facial movement, and larger and stronger muscles [97]. Injection doses for the masseter muscle are higher in the Asian population, and this may be due to slightly different standards of beauty, with Asians preferring a slimmer jaw line [27]. Since most of the AEs occur when higher doses have been injected, it is important to comprehend the adequate technique [54,56]. One interesting finding is that parotid gland hypertrophy injections for cosmetic reasons have only recently been reported in a consensus for Asians [28]. The treatment itself may be preferred in Asian countries where a bulky jaw is perceived as less attractive, and this can be caused by either a hypertrophic masseter muscle or hypertrophic parotid gland. The indications for BoNT are broadening in both esthetical and therapeutical fields. This may be due to adjunctive tools, such as US, that help in precise injection and monitoring of subsequent changes [65]. To date, BoNT has shown promising treatment modalities in many fields, and further research will render more accurate injection techniques and versatile applications.

5. Concluding Remarks

There has been a global rise in the demand for non-invasive procedures to help patients rejuvenate and appear youthful. BoNT is now the most performed esthetic procedure in the world with various types of BoNT that have different properties out in the market. More practitioners are using BoNT and demand appropriate guidelines so that injections using BoNT can be performed safely and effectively for the treatment of dynamic rhytides and hypertrophic structures. This paper is a narrative review of the consensus statements of expert practitioners and the various literature on the injection points and techniques, highlighting both the Asian and Caucasian population separately. This paper can serve as a practical illustrative guide and reference for optimal, safe injection areas and effective doses for application of BoNT in the face and oral and maxillofacial area. One limitation of this study was that a single author extracted the data and a systematic meta-analysis was not performed, and therefore the risk of bias was not investigated. Larger consensus statements and dose-ranging systematic studies comparing female to male, Caucasian to Asian, and younger to older patients should be conducted in the future.

Funding: This study was supported by the National Research Foundation of Korea (NRF) grant funded by the Korea government (MSIP; Ministry of Science, ICT & Future Planning) (No. 2017R1C1B-5018358) and by the Korea government (MSIT; Ministry of Science and ICT) (No. 2021R1F1A1049784).

Supplementary Materials: The following supporting information can be downloaded at: https://www.mdpi.com/article/10.3390/toxins15020082/s1, Table S1. List of 27 consensus recommendation papers retrieved for the literature review.

Institutional Review Board Statement: Not applicable.

Informed Consent Statement: Written informed consent was obtained from the patient to publish this paper.

Data Availability Statement: Not applicable.

Acknowledgments: The authors would like to thank Kyung Jun Park for his medical expertise and Byoung-Ae Kim for her technical assistance.

Conflicts of Interest: The author declares no conflict of interest.

Abbreviations

AE	Adverse effects
BoNT	Botulinum toxin
CSM	Corrugator supercilia muscle
DAO	Depressor anguli oris
DLI	Depressor labii inferioris
FM	Frontalis muscle
HAS	Human Serum Albumin
IM	Intramuscularly
U	International Unit
IV	Intravenously
L	Liquid
LLS	Levator labii superioris
LLSAN	Levator labii superioris alaeque nasi
NACL	Sodium chloride
NAPs	Neurotoxin-associated complexing proteins
OOc	Orbicularis oculi
OOr	Orbicularis oris
P	Powder
PO	Orally
q.s.	Quantum sufficit
US	Ultrasonography
Zmi	Zygomaticus minor
ZMj	Zygomaticus major
IP	Injection points
n	Number
F	Female
M	Male
Up	Upper
L	Lower
NR	Not reported

References

1. Liew, S.; Dart, A. Nonsurgical reshaping of the lower face. *Aesthet. Surg. J.* **2008**, *28*, 251–257. [CrossRef] [PubMed]
2. Swift, A.; Remington, K. BeautiPHIcation™: A global approach to facial beauty. *Clin. Plast. Surg.* **2011**, *38*, 347–377. [CrossRef]
3. Liew, S.; Wu, W.T.; Chan, H.H.; Ho, W.W.; Kim, H.J.; Goodman, G.J.; Peng, P.H.; Rogers, J.D. Consensus on changing trends, attitudes, and concepts of Asian beauty. *Aesthet. Plast. Surg.* **2016**, *40*, 193–201. [CrossRef]
4. Small, R. Botulinum toxin injection for facial wrinkles. *Am. Fam. Physician* **2014**, *90*, 168–175. [PubMed]
5. Zimbler, M.S.; Kokoska, M.S.; Thomas, J.R. Anatomy and pathophysiology of facial aging. *Facial Plast. Surg. Clin. N. Am.* **2001**, *9*, 179–187.
6. Gadhia, K.; Walmsley, A.D. Facial aesthetics: Is botulinum toxin treatment effective and safe? A systematic review of randomised controlled trials. *Br. Dent. J.* **2009**, *207*, E9; discussion 216–217. [CrossRef]
7. Phan, K.; Younessi, S.; Dubin, D.; Lin, M.J.; Khorasani, H. Emerging off-label esthetic uses of botulinum toxin in dermatology. *Dermatol. Ther.* **2022**, *35*, e15205. [CrossRef]
8. Frevert, J. Pharmaceutical, biological, and clinical properties of botulinum neurotoxin type A products. *Drugs R D* **2015**, *15*, 1–9. [CrossRef]
9. Alster, T.S.; Harrison, I.S. Alternative clinical indications of botulinum toxin. *Am. J. Clin. Derm.* **2020**, *21*, 855–880. [CrossRef]
10. Serrera-Figallo, M.A.; Ruiz-de-León-Hernández, G.; Torres-Lagares, D.; Castro-Araya, A.; Torres-Ferrerosa, O.; Hernández-Pacheco, E.; Gutierrez-Perez, J.L. Use of Botulinum Toxin in Orofacial Clinical Practice. *Toxins* **2020**, *12*, 112. [CrossRef]

11. Jankovic, J. Botulinum toxin: State of the art. *Mov. Disord.* **2017**, *32*, 1131–1138. [CrossRef] [PubMed]
12. Benecke, R. Clinical relevance of botulinum toxin immunogenicity. *BioDrugs* **2012**, *26*, e1–e9. [CrossRef] [PubMed]
13. Arnon, S.S.; Schechter, R.; Inglesby, T.V.; Henderson, D.A.; Bartlett, J.G.; Ascher, M.S.; Eitzen, E.; Fine, A.D.; Hauer, J.; Layton, M.; et al. Botulinum toxin as a biological weapon: Medical and public health management. *JAMA* **2001**, *285*, 1059–1070. [CrossRef]
14. Rosales, R.L.; Bigalke, H.; Dressler, D. Pharmacology of botulinum toxin: Differences between type A preparations. *Eur. J. Neurol.* **2006**, *13* (Suppl. S1), 2–10. [CrossRef] [PubMed]
15. Choudhury, S.; Baker, M.R.; Chatterjee, S.; Kumar, H. Botulinum Toxin: An Update on Pharmacology and Newer Products in Development. *Toxins* **2021**, *13*, 58. [CrossRef] [PubMed]
16. Zhang, S.; Masuyer, G.; Zhang, J.; Shen, Y.; Lundin, D.; Henriksson, L.; Miyashita, S.I.; Martínez-Carranza, M.; Dong, M.; Stenmark, P. Identification and characterization of a novel botulinum neurotoxin. *Nat. Commun.* **2017**, *8*, 14130. [CrossRef] [PubMed]
17. Carruthers, A.; Carruthers, J. Botulinum toxin type A. *J. Am. Acad. Derm.* **2005**, *53*, 284–290. [CrossRef] [PubMed]
18. Rao, A.K.; Sobel, J.; Chatham-Stephens, K.; Luquez, C. Clinical guidelines for diagnosis and treatment of botulism, 2021. *MMWR Recomm. Rep.* **2021**, *70*, 1–30. [CrossRef] [PubMed]
19. Jaspers, G.W.; Pijpe, J.; Jansma, J. The use of botulinum toxin type A in cosmetic facial procedures. *Int. J. Oral Maxillofac. Surg.* **2011**, *40*, 127–133. [CrossRef] [PubMed]
20. Kwon, K.H.; Shin, K.S.; Yeon, S.H.; Kwon, D.G. Application of botulinum toxin in maxillofacial field: Part I. Bruxism and square jaw. *Maxillofac. Plast. Reconstr. Surg.* **2019**, *41*, 38. [CrossRef] [PubMed]
21. Chang, C.S.; Bergeron, L.; Yu, C.C.; Chen, P.K.; Chen, Y.R. Mandible changes evaluated by computed tomography following Botulinum Toxin A injections in square-faced patients. *Aesthet. Plast. Surg.* **2011**, *35*, 452–455. [CrossRef] [PubMed]
22. Majid, O.W. Clinical use of botulinum toxins in oral and maxillofacial surgery. *Int. J. Oral Maxillofac. Surg.* **2010**, *39*, 197–207. [CrossRef] [PubMed]
23. Schantz, E.J.; Johnson, E.A. Properties and use of botulinum toxin and other microbial neurotoxins in medicine. *Microbiol. Rev.* **1992**, *56*, 80–99. [CrossRef] [PubMed]
24. Scott, A.B. Botulinum toxin injection into extraocular muscles as an alternative to strabismus surgery. *Ophthalmology* **1980**, *87*, 1044–1049. [CrossRef]
25. Carruthers, J.; Carruthers, A. Botulinum toxin in facial rejuvenation: An update. *Derm. Clin.* **2009**, *27*, 417–425. [CrossRef]
26. Muñoz Lora, V.R.M.; Del Bel Cury, A.A.; Jabbari, B.; Lacković, Z. Botulinum toxin type A in dental medicine. *J. Dent. Res.* **2019**, *98*, 1450–1457. [CrossRef]
27. Ahn, B.K.; Kim, Y.S.; Kim, H.J.; Rho, N.K.; Kim, H.S. Consensus recommendations on the aesthetic usage of botulinum toxin type A in Asians. *Derm. Surg.* **2013**, *39*, 1843–1860. [CrossRef]
28. Sundaram, H.; Huang, P.H.; Hsu, N.J.; Huh, C.H.; Wu, W.T.; Wu, Y.; Cassuto, D.; Kerscher, M.J.; Seo, K.K. Aesthetic applications of botulinum toxin A in Asians: An international, multidisciplinary, Pan-Asian consensus. *Plast. Reconstr. Surg. Glob. Open* **2016**, *4*, e872. [CrossRef]
29. Kapoor, K.M.; Chatrath, V.; Anand, C.; Shetty, R.; Chhabra, C.; Singh, K.; Vedamurthy, M.; Pai, J.; Sthalekar, B.; Sheth, R. Consensus recommendations for treatment strategies in Indians using botulinum toxin and Hyaluronic Acid fillers. *Plast. Reconstr. Surg. Glob. Open* **2017**, *5*, e1574. [CrossRef]
30. Wu, W.T.; Liew, S.; Chan, H.H.; Ho, W.W.; Supapannachart, N.; Lee, H.K.; Prasetyo, A.; Yu, J.N.; Rogers, J.D. Consensus on current injectable treatment strategies in the Asian face. *Aesthet. Plast. Surg.* **2016**, *40*, 202–214. [CrossRef]
31. Fagien, S.; Raspaldo, H. Facial rejuvenation with botulinum neurotoxin: An anatomical and experiential perspective. *J. Cosmet. Laser Ther.* **2007**, *9* (Suppl. S1), 23–31. [CrossRef] [PubMed]
32. Bertossi, D.; Cavallini, M.; Cirillo, P.; Piero Fundarò, S.; Quartucci, S.; Sciuto, C.; Tonini, D.; Trocchi, G.; Signorini, M. Italian consensus report on the aesthetic use of onabotulinum toxin A. *J. Cosmet. Derm.* **2018**, *17*, 719–730. [CrossRef] [PubMed]
33. Carruthers, J.; Fagien, S.; Matarasso, S.L. Consensus recommendations on the use of botulinum toxin type a in facial aesthetics. *Plast. Reconstr. Surg.* **2004**, *114* (Suppl. S6), 1s–22s. [CrossRef] [PubMed]
34. Carruthers, J.D.A.; Glogau, R.G.; Blitzer, A. Advances in facial rejuvenation: Botulinum toxin type a, hyaluronic acid dermal fillers, and combination therapies—Consensus recommendations. *Plast. Reconstr. Surg.* **2008**, *121* (Suppl. S5), 5s–30s. [CrossRef] [PubMed]
35. Carruthers, J.; Fournier, N.; Kerscher, M.; Ruiz-Avila, J.; Trindade de Almeida, A.R.; Kaeuper, G. The convergence of medicine and neurotoxins: A focus on botulinum toxin type A and its application in aesthetic medicine—A global, evidence-based botulinum toxin consensus education initiative: Part II: Incorporating botulinum toxin into aesthetic clinical practice. *Dermatol. Surg.* **2013**, *39 Pt 2*, 510–525.
36. Raspaldo, H.; Gassia, V.; Niforos, F.R.; Michaud, T. Global, 3-dimensional approach to natural rejuvenation: Part 1—Recommendations for volume restoration and the periocular area. *J. Cosmet. Derm.* **2012**, *11*, 279–289. [CrossRef]
37. Gassia, V.; Raspaldo, H.; Niforos, F.R.; Michaud, T. Global 3-dimensional approach to natural rejuvenation: Recommendations for perioral, nose, and ear rejuvenation. *J. Cosmet. Derm.* **2013**, *12*, 123–136. [CrossRef]

38. Raspaldo, H.; Niforos, F.R.; Gassia, V.; Dallara, J.M.; Bellity, P.; Baspeyras, M.; Belhaouari, L.; Group, C. Lower-face and neck antiaging treatment and prevention using onabotulinumtoxin A: The 2010 multidisciplinary French consensus—Part 2. *J. Cosmet. Dermatol.* **2011**, *10*, 131–149. [CrossRef]
39. Raspaldo, H.; Baspeyras, M.; Bellity, P.; Dallara, J.M.; Gassia, V.; Niforos, F.R.; Belhaouari, L. Upper- and mid-face anti-aging treatment and prevention using onabotulinumtoxin A: The 2010 multidisciplinary French consensus—Part 1. *J. Cosmet. Dermatol.* **2011**, *10*, 36–50. [CrossRef]
40. Ascher, B.; Talarico, S.; Cassuto, D.; Escobar, S.; Hexsel, D.; Jaén, P.; Monheit, G.D.; Rzany, B.; Viel, M. International consensus recommendations on the aesthetic usage of botulinum toxin type A (Speywood Unit)—Part II: Wrinkles on the middle and lower face, neck and chest. *J. Eur. Acad. Derm. Venereol.* **2010**, *24*, 1285–1295. [CrossRef]
41. Kane, M.; Donofrio, L.; Ascher, B.; Hexsel, D.; Monheit, G.; Rzany, B.; Weiss, R. Expanding the use of neurotoxins in facial aesthetics: A consensus panel's assessment and recommendations. *J. Drugs Derm.* **2010**, *9* (Suppl. S1), s7–s22, quiz s23–s25.
42. Ascher, B.; Talarico, S.; Cassuto, D.; Escobar, S.; Hexsel, D.; Jaén, P.; Monheit, G.D.; Rzany, B.; Viel, M. International consensus recommendations on the aesthetic usage of botulinum toxin type A (Speywood Unit)—Part I: Upper facial wrinkles. *J. Eur. Acad. Derm. Venereol.* **2010**, *24*, 1278–1284. [CrossRef] [PubMed]
43. Yutskovskaya, Y.; Gubanova, E.; Khrustaleva, I.; Atamanov, V.; Saybel, A.; Parsagashvili, E.; Dmitrieva, I.; Sanchez, E.; Lapatina, N.; Korolkova, T.; et al. IncobotulinumtoxinA in aesthetics: Russian multidisciplinary expert consensus recommendations. *Clin. Cosmet. Investig. Derm.* **2015**, *8*, 297–306.
44. Maas, C.; Kane, M.A.; Bucay, V.W.; Allen, S.; Applebaum, D.J.; Baumann, L.; Cox, S.E.; Few, J.W.; Joseph, J.H.; Lorenc, Z.P.; et al. Current aesthetic use of abobotulinumtoxinA in clinical practice: An evidence-based consensus review. *Aesthet. Surg. J.* **2012**, *32* (Suppl. S1), 8s–29s. [CrossRef]
45. Imhof, M.; Podda, M.; Sommer, B. S1 guideline aesthetic botulinum toxin therapy. *J. Dtsch. Derm. Ges.* **2013**, *11*, e1–e13. [CrossRef]
46. Lorenc, Z.P.; Kenkel, J.M.; Fagien, S.; Hirmand, H.; Nestor, M.S.; Sclafani, A.P.; Sykes, J.M.; Waldorf, H.A. Consensus panel's assessment and recommendations on the use of 3 botulinum toxin type A products in facial aesthetics. *Aesthet. Surg. J.* **2013**, *33* (Suppl. S1), 35s–40s.
47. Sundaram, H.; Signorini, M.; Liew, S.; Trindade de Almeida, A.R.; Wu, Y.; Vieira Braz, A.; Fagien, S.; Goodman, G.J.; Monheit, G.; Raspaldo, H. Global Aesthetics Consensus: Botulinum Toxin Type A—Evidence-Based Review, Emerging Concepts, and Consensus Recommendations for Aesthetic Use, Including Updates on Complications. *Plast. Reconstr. Surg.* **2016**, *137*, 518e–529e. [CrossRef]
48. Sundaram, H.; Liew, S.; Signorini, M.; Vieira Braz, A.; Fagien, S.; Swift, A.; De Boulle, K.L.; Raspaldo, H.; Trindade de Almeida, A.R.; Monheit, G. Global aesthetics consensus: Hyaluronic Acid billers and botulinum toxin type A-recommendations for combined treatment and optimizing outcomes in diverse patient populations. *Plast. Reconstr. Surg.* **2016**, *137*, 1410–1423. [CrossRef]
49. De Maio, M.; Swift, A.; Signorini, M.; Fagien, S. Facial assessment and injection guide for botulinum toxin and injectable Hyaluronic Acid fillers: Focus on the upper Face. *Plast. Reconstr. Surg.* **2017**, *140*, 265e–276e. [CrossRef]
50. De Maio, M.; DeBoulle, K.; Braz, A.; Rohrich, R.J. Facial Assessment and Injection Guide for Botulinum toxin and injectable Hyaluronic Acid fillers: Focus on the midface. *Plast. Reconstr. Surg.* **2017**, *140*, 540e–550e. [CrossRef]
51. De Maio, M.; Wu, W.T.L.; Goodman, G.J.; Monheit, G. Facial assessment and injection guide for botulinum toxin and injectable Hyaluronic Acid fillers: Focus on the lower face. *Plast. Reconstr. Surg.* **2017**, *140*, 393e–404e. [CrossRef] [PubMed]
52. Kaminer, M.S.; Cox, S.E.; Fagien, S.; Kaufman, J.; Lupo, M.P.; Shamban, A. Re-examining the optimal use of neuromodulators and the changing landscape: A consensus panel update. *J. Drugs Derm.* **2020**, *19*, s5–s15.
53. Signorini, M.; Piero Fundarò, S.; Bertossi, D.; Cavallini, M.; Cirillo, P.; Natuzzi, G.; Quartucci, S.; Sciuto, C.; Patalano, M.; Trocchi, G. OnabotulinumtoxinA from lines to facial reshaping: A new Italian consensus report. *J. Cosmet. Derm.* **2022**, *21*, 550–563. [CrossRef] [PubMed]
54. Camargo, C.P.; Xia, J.; Costa, C.S.; Gemperli, R.; Tatini, M.D.; Bulsara, M.K.; Riera, R. Botulinum toxin type A for facial wrinkles. *Cochrane Database Syst. Rev.* **2021**, *7*, 011301.
55. Janes, L.E.; Connor, L.M.; Moradi, A.; Alghoul, M. Current use of cosmetic toxins to improve facial aesthetics. *Plast. Reconstr. Surg.* **2021**, *147*, 644e–657e. [CrossRef]
56. Kim, H.-J.; Seo, K.K.; Lee, H.-K.; Kim, J. Clinical anatomy for botulinum toxin injection. In *Clinical Anatomy of the Face for Filler and Botulinum Toxin Injection*; Springer: Singapore, 2016; pp. 55–92.
57. Klein, A.W. Complications, adverse reactions, and insights with the use of botulinum toxin. *Derm. Surg.* **2003**, *29*, 549–556.
58. Kwon, K.H.; Shin, K.S.; Yeon, S.H.; Kwon, D.G. Application of botulinum toxin in maxillofacial field: Part II. Wrinkle, intraoral ulcer, and cranio-maxillofacial pain. *Maxillofac. Plast. Reconstr. Surg.* **2019**, *41*, 42. [CrossRef]
59. Pirazzini, M.; Rossetto, O.; Eleopra, R.; Montecucco, C. Botulinum Neurotoxins: Biology, Pharmacology, and Toxicology. *Pharm. Rev.* **2017**, *69*, 200–235. [CrossRef]
60. Frevert, J.; Ahn, K.Y.; Park, M.Y.; Sunga, O. Comparison of botulinum neurotoxin type A formulations in Asia. *Clin. Cosmet. Investig. Dermatol.* **2018**, *11*, 327–331. [CrossRef]
61. Solish, N.; Carruthers, J.; Kaufman, J.; Rubio, R.G.; Gross, T.M.; Gallagher, C.J. Overview of DaxibotulinumtoxinA for injection: A novel formulation of botulinum toxin type A. *Drugs* **2021**, *81*, 2091–2101. [CrossRef]

62. Inoue, K.; Fujinaga, Y.; Watanabe, T.; Ohyama, T.; Takeshi, K.; Moriishi, K.; Nakajima, H.; Inoue, K.; Oguma, K. Molecular composition of Clostridium botulinum type A progenitor toxins. *Infect. Immun.* **1996**, *64*, 1589–1594. [CrossRef] [PubMed]
63. Goodnough, M.C.; Johnson, E.A. Stabilization of botulinum toxin type A during lyophilization. *Appl. Environ. Microbiol.* **1992**, *58*, 3426–3428. [CrossRef] [PubMed]
64. Dover, J.S.; Monheit, G.; Greener, M.; Pickett, A. Botulinum toxin in aesthetic medicine: Myths and realities. *Dermatol. Surg.* **2018**, *44*, 249–260. [CrossRef] [PubMed]
65. Kim, H.-J.; Youn, K.-H.; Kim, J.-S.; Kim, Y.S.; Hong, S.O.; Na, J. US applications in botulinum toxin injection procedures. In *Ultrasonographic Anatomy of the Face and Neck for Minimally Invasive Procedures: An Anatomic Guideline for Ultrasonographic-Guided Procedures*; Springer: Singapore, 2021; pp. 215–241.
66. Kim, H.-J.; Youn, K.-H.; Kim, J.-S.; Kim, Y.S.; Hong, S.O.; Na, J. General US anatomy of the face and neck. In *Ultrasonographic Anatomy of the Face and Neck for Minimally Invasive Procedures: An Anatomic Guideline for Ultrasonographic-Guided Procedures*; Springer: Singapore, 2021; pp. 25–73.
67. Gart, M.S.; Gutowski, K.A. Overview of botulinum toxins for aesthetic uses. *Clin. Plast. Surg.* **2016**, *43*, 459–471. [CrossRef]
68. Kokich, V.O.; Kokich, V.G.; Kiyak, H.A. Perceptions of dental professionals and laypersons to altered dental esthetics: Asymmetric and symmetric situations. *Am. J. Orthod. Dentofac. Orthop.* **2006**, *130*, 141–151. [CrossRef] [PubMed]
69. Hong, S.O.; Baek, S.H.; Choi, J.Y. Physical therapy for smile improvement after orthognathic Surgery. *J. Craniofac. Surg.* **2017**, *28*, 422–426. [CrossRef]
70. Mazzuco, R.; Hexsel, D. Gummy smile and botulinum toxin: A new approach based on the gingival exposure area. *J. Am. Acad. Derm.* **2010**, *63*, 1042–1051. [CrossRef]
71. Hwang, W.S.; Hur, M.S.; Hu, K.S.; Song, W.C.; Koh, K.S.; Baik, H.S.; Kim, S.T.; Kim, H.J.; Lee, K.J. Surface anatomy of the lip elevator muscles for the treatment of gummy smile using botulinum toxin. *Angle Orthod.* **2009**, *79*, 70–77. [CrossRef] [PubMed]
72. Kundu, N.; Kothari, R.; Shah, N.; Sandhu, S.; Tripathy, D.M.; Galadari, H.; Gold, M.H.; Goldman, M.P.; Kassir, M.; Schepler, H.; et al. Efficacy of botulinum toxin in masseter muscle hypertrophy for lower face contouring. *J. Cosmet. Derm.* **2022**, *21*, 1849–1856. [CrossRef] [PubMed]
73. Kroumpouzos, G.; Kassir, M.; Gupta, M.; Patil, A.; Goldust, M. Complications of botulinum toxin, A. An update review. *J. Cosmet. Derm.* **2021**, *20*, 1585–1590. [CrossRef]
74. Park, H.J.; Hong, S.O.; Kim, H.M.; Oh, W.; Kim, H.J. Positional deformation of the parotid gland: Application to minimally invasive procedures. *Clin. Anat.* **2022**, *35*, 1147–1151. [CrossRef] [PubMed]
75. Teymoortash, A.; Sommer, F.; Mandic, R.; Schulz, S.; Bette, M.; Aumüller, G.; Werner, J.A. Intraglandular application of botulinum toxin leads to structural and functional changes in rat acinar cells. *Br. J. Pharm.* **2007**, *152*, 161–167. [CrossRef] [PubMed]
76. Ondo, W.G.; Hunter, C.; Moore, W. A double-blind placebo-controlled trial of botulinum toxin B for sialorrhea in Parkinson's disease. *Neurology* **2004**, *62*, 37–40. [CrossRef] [PubMed]
77. Jackson, C.E.; Gronseth, G.; Rosenfeld, J.; Barohn, R.J.; Dubinsky, R.; Simpson, C.B.; McVey, A.; Kittrell, P.P.; King, R.; Herbelin, L. Randomized double-blind study of botulinum toxin type B for sialorrhea in ALS patients. *Muscle Nerve* **2009**, *39*, 137–143. [CrossRef]
78. Kim, H.-J.; Youn, K.-H.; Kim, J.-S.; Kim, Y.S.; Hong, S.O.; Na, J. US Applications in filler injection procedures. In *Ultrasonographic Anatomy of the Face and Neck for Minimally Invasive Procedures: An Anatomic Guideline for Ultrasonographic-Guided Procedures*; Springer: Singapore, 2021; pp. 243–264.
79. Kim, H.-J.; Youn, K.-H.; Kim, J.-S.; Kim, Y.S.; Hong, S.O.; Na, J. US applications in thread lifting procedures. In *Ultrasonographic Anatomy of the Face and Neck for Minimally Invasive Procedures: An Anatomic Guideline for Ultrasonographic-Guided Procedures*; Springer: Singapore, 2021; pp. 265–274.
80. Lee, H.J.; Kim, J.S.; Youn, K.H.; Lee, J.; Kim, H.J. Ultras.sound-guided botulinum neurotoxin type A injection for correcting asymmetrical smiles. *Aesthet. Surg. J.* **2018**, *38*, 130–134. [CrossRef]
81. Kim, D.; Park, J.H.; Favero, V.; Mah, J.; Jung, Y.S.; Kim, S.T. Effect of botulinum toxin injection on asymmetric lower face with chin deviation. *Toxins* **2020**, *12*, 456. [CrossRef]
82. Wollina, U.; Konrad, H. Managing adverse events associated with botulinum toxin type A: A focus on cosmetic procedures. *Am. J. Clin. Derm.* **2005**, *6*, 141–150. [CrossRef]
83. Zargaran, D.; Zoller, F.; Zargaran, A.; Rahman, E.; Woollard, A.; Weyrich, T.; Mosahebi, A. Complications of cosmetic botulinum toxin A injections to the upper face: A systematic review and meta-analysis. *Aesthet. Surg. J.* **2022**, *42*, 327–336. [CrossRef]
84. Sethi, N.; Singh, S.; DeBoulle, K.; Rahman, E. A review of Complications due to the use of botulinum toxin A for cosmetic indications. *Aesthet. Plast. Surg.* **2021**, *45*, 1210–1220. [CrossRef]
85. Galadari, H.; Galadari, I.; Smit, R.; Prygova, I.; Redaelli, A. Use of AbobotulinumtoxinA for cosmetic treatments in the neck, and middle and lower areas of the face: A systematic review. *Toxins* **2021**, *13*, 169. [CrossRef]
86. Wang, L.; Sun, Y.; Yang, W.; Lindo, P.; Singh, B.R. Type A botulinum neurotoxin complex proteins differentially modulate host response of neuronal cells. *Toxicon* **2014**, *82*, 52–60. [CrossRef]
87. Wee, S.Y.; Park, E.S. Immunogenicity of botulinum toxin. *Arch. Plast. Surg.* **2022**, *49*, 12–18. [CrossRef] [PubMed]
88. Albrecht, P.; Jansen, A.; Lee, J.I.; Moll, M.; Ringelstein, M.; Rosenthal, D.; Bigalke, H.; Aktas, O.; Hartung, H.P.; Hefter, H. High prevalence of neutralizing antibodies after long-term botulinum neurotoxin therapy. *Neurology* **2019**, *92*, e48–e54. [CrossRef] [PubMed]

89. Wu, Y.; Wang, G.; Li, C.; Mao, C.; Lei, X.; Lee, E. Safety and Efficacy of OnabotulinumtoxinA for Treatment of Crow's Feet Lines in Chinese Subjects. *Plast. Reconstr. Surg. Glob. Open* **2019**, *7*, e2079. [CrossRef] [PubMed]
90. Moers-Carpi, M.; Dirschka, T.; Feller-Heppt, G.; Hilton, S.; Hoffmann, K.; Philipp-Dormston, W.G.; Rütter, A.; Tan, K.; Chapman, M.A.; Fulford-Smith, A. A randomised, double-blind comparison of 20 units of onabotulinumtoxinA with 30 units of incobotulinumtoxinA for glabellar lines. *J. Cosmet. Laser Ther.* **2012**, *14*, 296–303. [CrossRef] [PubMed]
91. Ascher, B.; Kestemont, P.; Boineau, D.; Bodokh, I.; Stein, A.; Heckmann, M.; Dendorfer, M.; Pavicic, T.; Volteau, M.; Tse, A.; et al. Liquid formulation of AbobotulinumtoxinA exhibits a favorable efficacy and safety profile in moderate to severe glabellar Lines: A randomized, double-blind, placebo- and active comparator-controlled trial. *Aesthet. Surg. J.* **2018**, *38*, 183–191. [CrossRef]
92. Carruthers, A.; Carruthers, J. A single-center, dose-comparison, pilot study of botulinum neurotoxin type A in female patients with upper facial rhytids: Safety and efficacy. *J. Am. Acad. Derm.* **2009**, *60*, 972–979. [CrossRef]
93. Kerscher, M.; Rzany, B.; Prager, W.; Turnbull, C.; Trevidic, P.; Inglefield, C. Efficacy and safety of IncobotulinumtoxinA in the Treatment of Upper Facial Lines: Results From a randomized, double-blind, placebo-controlled, phase III study. *Derm. Surg.* **2015**, *41*, 1149–1157. [CrossRef]
94. Cheon, H.I.; Jung, N.; Won, C.H.; Kim, B.J.; Lee, Y.W. Efficacy and safety of Prabotulinumtoxin A and Onabotulinumtoxin A for Crow's feet: A phase 3, multicenter, randomized, double-blind, split-face study. *Derm. Surg.* **2019**, *45*, 1610–1619. [CrossRef]
95. Carruthers, J.; Carruthers, A.; Monheit, G.D.; Davis, P.G. Multicenter, randomized, parallel-group study of onabotulinumtoxinA and hyaluronic acid dermal fillers (24-mg/ml smooth, cohesive gel) alone and in combination for lower facial rejuvenation: Satisfaction and patient-reported outcomes. *Dermatol. Surg.* **2010**, *36* (Suppl. S4), 2135–2145. [CrossRef]
96. Cohen, J.L.; Dayan, S.H.; Cox, S.E.; Yalamanchili, R.; Tardie, G. OnabotulinumtoxinA dose-ranging study for hyperdynamic perioral lines. *Derm. Surg.* **2012**, *38*, 1497–1505. [CrossRef] [PubMed]
97. Kandhari, R.; Imran, A.; Sethi, N.; Rahman, E.; Mosahebi, A. Onabotulinumtoxin Type A Dosage for upper face expression lines in males: A systematic review of current recommendations. *Aesthet. Surg. J.* **2021**, *41*, 1439–1453. [CrossRef] [PubMed]

toxins

MDPI

Review

Neurophysiological Basis of Deep Brain Stimulation and Botulinum Neurotoxin Injection for Treating Oromandibular Dystonia

Hitoshi Maezawa [1,2,*], Masayuki Hirata [2] and Kazuya Yoshida [3]

1 Faculty of Rehabilitation, Kansai Medical University, Uyama-higashi 18-89, Hirakata 573-1136, Japan
2 Department of Neurological Diagnosis and Restoration, Graduate School of Medicine, Osaka University, Yamadaoka 2-2, Suita 565-0871, Japan
3 Department of Oral and Maxillofacial Surgery, National Hospital Organization, Kyoto Medical Center, 1-1 Mukaihata-cho, Fukakusa, Fushimi-ku, Kyoto 612-8555, Japan
* Correspondence: maezawah@makino.kmu.ac.jp

Abstract: Oromandibular dystonia (OMD) induces severe motor impairments, such as masticatory disturbances, dysphagia, and dysarthria, resulting in a serious decline in quality of life. Non-invasive brain-imaging techniques such as electroencephalography (EEG) and magnetoencephalography (MEG) are powerful approaches that can elucidate human cortical activity with high temporal resolution. Previous studies with EEG and MEG have revealed that movements in the stomatognathic system are regulated by the bilateral central cortex. Recently, in addition to the standard therapy of botulinum neurotoxin (BoNT) injection into the affected muscles, bilateral deep brain stimulation (DBS) has been applied for the treatment of OMD. However, some patients' OMD symptoms do not improve sufficiently after DBS, and they require additional BoNT therapy. In this review, we provide an overview of the unique central spatiotemporal processing mechanisms in these regions in the bilateral cortex using EEG and MEG, as they relate to the sensorimotor functions of the stomatognathic system. Increased knowledge regarding the neurophysiological underpinnings of the stomatognathic system will improve our understanding of OMD and other movement disorders, as well as aid the development of potential novel approaches such as combination treatment with BoNT injection and DBS or non-invasive cortical current stimulation therapies.

Keywords: oromandibular dystonia; botulinum neurotoxin; stomatognathic function; deep brain stimulation; sensorimotor function; magnetoencephalography; electroencephalography; motor function; globus pallidus

Key Contribution: The uncertain effects of deep brain stimulation (DBS) on oromandibular dystonia may, in part, be explained by the unique characteristics of the bilateral central regulation of sensorimotor functions in the stomatognathic system. An improved understanding of the central mechanisms related to stomatognathic functions will promote the development of new approaches, such as combination treatment with botulinum neurotoxin injection and DBS or non-invasive cortical current stimulation therapies.

Citation: Maezawa, H.; Hirata, M.; Yoshida, K. Neurophysiological Basis of Deep Brain Stimulation and Botulinum Neurotoxin Injection for Treating Oromandibular Dystonia. *Toxins* **2022**, *14*, 751. https://doi.org/10.3390/toxins14110751

Received: 10 October 2022
Accepted: 1 November 2022
Published: 2 November 2022

1. Introduction

The stomatognathic system is an anatomic and functional unit comprising the mandible, maxilla, dental arches, teeth, temporomandibular joint, masticatory muscles, surrounding nerves and vessels, and salivary glands. The stomatognathic system plays important roles in a variety of critical motor functions, including mastication, swallowing, speech production, and respiration. Focal dystonia in the stomatognathic system induces severe motor dysfunction that negatively affects quality of life via factors such as masticatory disturbances, limited mouth opening, dysphagia, and dysarthria caused by involuntary movements in the stomatognathic system [1–3].

Dystonia is characterized by sustained or intermittent muscle contractions that produce involuntary, unwanted, and often repetitive movements, postural changes, or both [4]. Focal dystonia includes blepharospasm (eyelids), cervical dystonia (neck), writer's cramp, musician's cramp (hand and arm), and oromandibular dystonia (OMD) [5]. OMD is a focal type of dystonia that involves the masticatory, lower facial, lingual, or orbicularis oris muscles [1–3,6]. Clinically, OMD presents as dystonia during jaw opening or closing, jaw deviation, jaw protrusion, lingual dystonia, lip dystonia, or a combination of these abnormal movements [7].

When OMD occurs in conjunction with blepharospasm, it is usually referred to as Meige syndrome. Meige syndrome, which was first described by Henri Meige in 1910, is cranial dystonia characterized by the combination of upper and lower cranial involvement and including blepharospasm and OMD [8]. In Meige's syndrome, there is progressive worsening of blepharospasm with the spread of symptoms to involve the oromandibular, cervical, and limb muscles; however, the symptoms spread earliest and greatest in the oromandibular muscles [9–11].

A recent multicenter study conducted among Institutions across seven countries found that OMD had a prevalence of 8.7% among all types of focal dystonia, making it one of the less prevalent subtypes of this neurological disorder [12]. The overall prevalence of primary dystonia was calculated as 16.4 per 100,000 cases in a meta-analysis [13], and that of OMD was estimated at 6.8 per 100,000 cases [14]. Another study reported an estimated OMD prevalence rate of 0.33 per 100,000 cases [15]. However, most of the studies evaluated relatively few patients with OMD. A recent epidemiologic study of 144 patients with OMD reported an estimated prevalence of 9.8 per 100,000 cases, suggesting that OMD is as common as cervical dystonia or blepharospasm [16].

Botulinum neurotoxin (BoNT) injection represents a standard therapy for focal dystonia, including cases of OMD [3,17]. BoNT is injected into the target muscles exhibiting disordered movements where it blocks acetylcholine release at the neuromuscular junction (NMJ). Proper muscle identification, dose selection, and management of patient expectations are required to ensure that BoNT injection is both safe and effective in patients with OMD [3], since stomatognathic functions are performed by various bilateral muscles in the stomatognathic system that differ in size and tension. Moreover, since each muscle of the stomatognathic system is controlled by the bilateral cortex through the corticobulbar tract and certain cranial nerves (CNs (CN V, VII, X, XII)), identifying the neurophysiological and neuroanatomical basis of sensorimotor functions in the stomatognathic system remains essential.

In addition to BoNT injection, deep brain stimulation (DBS) represents an optional therapy for focal dystonia in the limbs [18]. The main target of conventional DBS is the internal segment of the unilateral globus pallidus (GPi). DBS of the unilateral GPi improves symptoms of disordered movement on the contralateral side, based on the principle that unilateral movements in the limbs are regulated by the contralateral sides of the central regions via the corticospinal tract (Figure 1). However, the application of DBS for OMD has been limited, and evidence regarding its clinical utility in these patients is still considered preliminary.

Several case reports from the past two decades have described the use of DBS of the bilateral Gpi for the treatment of lingual dystonia [19–22]. This bilateral approach is based on the neurophysiological principle that tongue movements are regulated by the bilateral central regions through the corticobulbar tract, which differs from the contralateral regulation of the limbs (Figure 1). The uncertain effects of DBS on OMD may, in part, be explained by the unique characteristics of the bilateral central regulation of sensorimotor functions in the stomatognathic system. To establish effective treatments targeting the central regions, including DBS, further research is required to elucidate the neurophysiological basis and central mechanisms related to stomatognathic functions.

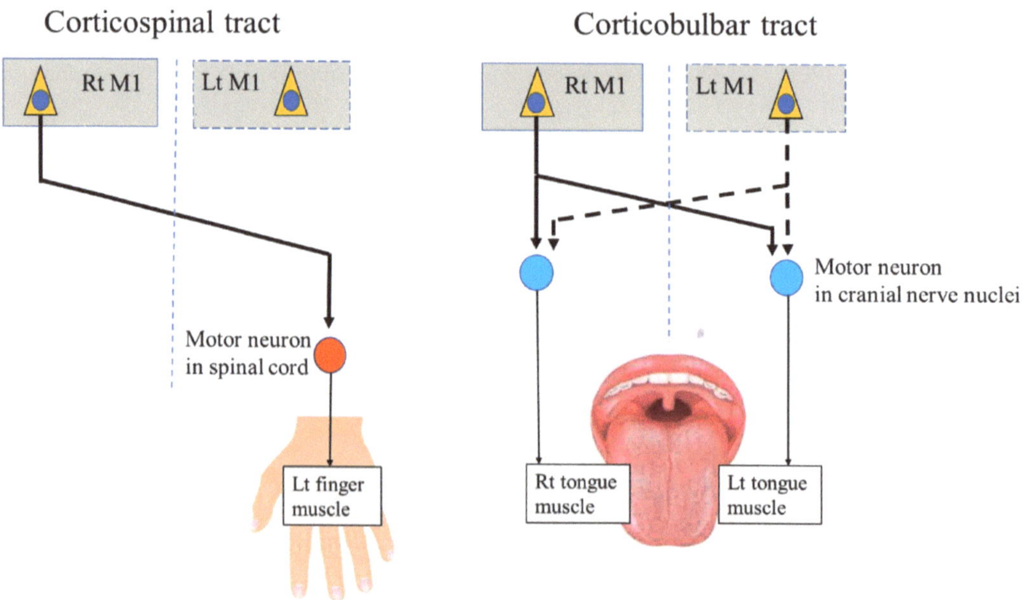

Figure 1. Corticospinal tract and corticobulbar tract. M1: primary motor cortex, Rt: right, Lt: left.

Recent advances in non-invasive electromagnetic physiological techniques, such as electroencephalography (EEG) and magnetoencephalography (MEG), have enabled the investigation of cortical mechanisms in humans with high temporal resolution. In particular, MEG is advantageous owing to its high spatial resolution given that the magnetic permeability of biological tissues is nearly identical to that of empty space; thus, the magnetic field is not distorted by the scalp or skull [23].

In this review, we present an overview of the unique central mechanisms of bilateral spatiotemporal processing associated with the sensorimotor functions of the stomatognathic system. These mechanisms have been demonstrated in MEG/EEG studies using multiple parameters for analysis, including somatosensory evoked fields/potentials (SEFs/SEPs), movement-related cortical fields/potentials (MRCFs/MRCPs), and cortico-muscular/cortico-kinematic coherence (CMC/CKC). We also discuss the pathophysiological characteristics of typical cases of hand dystonia, such as writer's cramp and OMD, as demonstrated using EEG and MEG. Finally, we identify current problems and future directions in OMD treatment.

2. Neural Pathways from the Primary Motor Cortex (M1) to Stomatognathic Systems

In the human primary motor cortex (M1), the cortical representations of various body parts are organized in the form of the "classical homunculus" [24]. In general, the homunculus resembles an upside-down map of each body part, in which the stomatognathic systems are closer to the lateral sulcus than the upper and lower extremities. The area of the M1 that represents the stomatognathic system is widely distributed relative to its actual size in the body [24], suggesting a rich innervation of these areas.

Anatomically, each muscle of the stomatognathic system receives innervation from the bilateral M1 through the corticobulbar tract, which terminates in motor neurons within the CN nuclei (Figure 1). In contrast, the muscles of the upper and lower limbs are predominantly innervated by the contralateral cortex through the corticospinal tract, which terminates in motor neurons within the spinal cord (Figure 1). Indeed, a previous study in patients with epilepsy showed that direct unilateral cortical stimulation of the M1 areas for the oral and upper limb muscles induced bilateral oral movements but unilateral limb movements [24].

The stomatognathic system is composed of various muscles, including the tongue muscles, orbicularis oris, and masticatory muscles responsible for jaw closing (masseter, temporalis, and medial pterygoid) and opening (inferior head of lateral pterygoid, anterior belly of digastric, geniohyoid, and mylohyoid). All the muscles of the tongue are innervated by the hypoglossal nerve (CN XII), except for the palatoglossal muscles, which are innervated by the vagus nerve (CN X). Masticatory muscles are innervated by the trigeminal nerve (CN V), except for the posterior bellies of the digastric muscles, which are innervated by the facial nerve (CN VII). The orbicularis oris muscle is innervated by the facial nerve (CN VII).

Moreover, bilateral innervation contributes to somatosensory sensations in the stomatognathic system. Somatosensory information from the tongue is transmitted by the mandibular branch of the trigeminal nerve (CN V) (anterior two-thirds of the tongue), glossopharyngeal nerve (CN IX) (posterior one-third of the tongue), and vagus nerve (posterior part of the tongue root) (CN X). Somatosensory information from the soft palate, teeth, gingiva, face, and lips is transmitted by the mandibular or maxillary branches of the trigeminal nerve (CN V). Proprioceptive sensations from the tongue muscle are transmitted by the hypoglossal nerve (CN XII) and its rich innervation of the related muscle spindles. Proprioceptive sensations from the masticatory muscles are mainly transmitted by the trigeminal nerve (CN V) for jaw-closing muscles, as the jaw-closing muscles have many more muscle spindles than the jaw-opening muscles [25].

3. Bilateral Brain Activation Related to Stomatognathic Functions

A previous study involving non-invasive, whole-head MEG successfully identified the classical homunculus in the primary somatosensory cortex following tactile stimulation of multiple points on the human body [26]. Cortical representations of oromandibular areas are widely distributed in the primary sensorimotor cortex relative to their actual size in the human body [26]. In this section, we describe in detail the unique central mechanisms of bilateral spatiotemporal information processing involved in the sensorimotor functions of the stomatognathic system, as demonstrated using MEG/EEG.

3.1. Movement-Related Cortical Fields and Potentials

In early studies, researchers observed slowly increasing cortical fields over the contralateral hemisphere before the onset of voluntary unilateral movements of a finger, which they termed MRCFs [27,28]. Cheyne et al. [29] first reported MRCFs associated with repetitive tongue protrusion in a patient using a seven-channel MEG system to record from the left hemisphere. Nakasato et al. [30] demonstrated whole-head MRCFs for tongue protrusion in five healthy volunteers, using a trigger signal that was detected when the tip of the tongue reached the anterior region of the palate. They reported that the peak magnitude of the MRCFs was derived from the areas of the bilateral M1 region representing the tongue. A recent MEG study investigated the characteristics of bilateral MRCFs before and after voluntary self-paced tongue movements, using surface electromyography (EMG) from the tongue [31]. As reported in previous MRCF studies of finger movement [27,28,32], three components were detected in response to tongue movement: the readiness field (RF), motor field (MF), and movement-evoked field (MEF). Slowly increasing RF components were observed bilaterally before the onset of movement, peaking in MFs around the onset of movement. The MF component appeared after the pre-movement RF component and originated from part of the primary motor area (M1) representing the tongue. The MEF component, which appears after movement onset and originates from the bilateral primary somatosensory area (S1), may reflect proprioceptive feedback from the tongue during voluntary tongue movement. These results suggest that the bilateral M1 and S1 are involved in the preparation and execution of tongue movements [31].

MRCPs are slowly increasing cortical shifts in negative potentials that occur prior to voluntary movements, as demonstrated using EEG [33]. In an EEG study of MRCPs related to jaw movement, a previous study [33] reported a slowly increasing negative potential originating 1.5–2 s before EMG onset, known as the Bereitschaftspotential (BP) [34,35]. The BP, also called the readiness potential, is a measure of brain activity in the motor cortex and supplementary motor area leading up to voluntary muscle movement. The maximum BP occurred over the vertex region, and the negative slope (NS′) occurred approximately 300–700 ms before EMG onset. The authors reported that BP/NS′ amplitudes at the onset of movement differed significantly among open, closed, and lateral movements. The MRCPs at mouth opening and closing were symmetrically distributed, whereas those at lateral movements were predominant over the hemisphere ipsilateral to the direction of movement.

In an MEG study of jaw movement in five healthy volunteers [36], RFs were observed bilaterally, starting around 860 and 600 ms prior to the onset of masseter and digastric EMGs, respectively, and gradually increasing in magnitude until peaking within 100 ms before EMG onset. In all participants, the equivalent current dipoles generating the RFs accompanying jaw-opening movements were located in the bilateral M1 areas representing the jaw. These results suggest that MRCF/MRCP recordings provide a means for exploring the spatiotemporal characteristics of the sensorimotor cortex before and after voluntary movements in the stomatognathic system.

3.2. Cortico-Muscular Coherence and Cortico-Kinematic Coherence during Voluntary Movements

CMC analyses can aid in evaluating oscillatory functional connections between the motor cortex and corresponding peripheral muscles during sustained muscle contraction [37,38]. The CMC in the β-frequency band (β-CMC) during the sustained unilateral movements of a finger mainly represents the descending motor commands from the M1 to the contralateral finger muscle through corticospinal pathways [38]. In our previous MEG study [39], the CMC of the tongue was detected at two different frequency bands (the β-band and a low-frequency band at 2–10 Hz) over both hemispheres for each side of the tongue during isometric tongue protrusion [39,40]. The β-CMC for the tongue mainly reflects the descending motor commands from each side of the M1 to both sides of the tongue, with contralateral dominance through hypoglossal motoneuron pools (Figure 2). Moreover, the somatotopic organization of the tongue and finger regions in the M1 allows for differentiation of the cortical source locations of the β-CMC for the tongue and finger [39]. In contrast to β-CMC, CMC in the low-frequency band (low-CMC) reflects oscillatory coupling related to proprioceptive feedback from the tongue muscles to the bilateral S1 [40]. This pattern of central regulation with oscillatory activity in two frequency bands is a unique characteristic of stomatognathic functions, since a stable low-CMC is not detected during finger movements.

CKC methods are used to quantify the coupling between MEG signals and finger kinematics, which are measured using an accelerometer during repetitive, rhythmic, or voluntary finger movements [41]. A recent MEG study has demonstrated that CKC data mainly reflect proprioceptive sensory feedback from the peripheral muscles to S1 [42]. However, applying conventional CKC to stomatognathic systems is difficult, as magnetic accelerometer devices can easily produce excessive magnetic artefacts due to the short distance between the brain and stomatognathic systems. To overcome this limitation, a recent MEG study successfully utilized a deep-learning-assisted motion capture system, in which the CKC was detected during rhythmic tongue movements at the frequency peaks of movement or its harmonics, based on signals in the bilateral primary sensorimotor cortex representing the tongue regions [43]. This combination of CKC and deep learning-assisted motion capture has the advantage of being noise-, movement-, and risk-free, particularly in the oral regions, because recording devices are not placed in the orofacial region. As the tongue muscles and those responsible for closing the jaw are rich in muscle spindles [25], the CKC approach may help to reveal the central proprioceptive mechanisms of the stomatognathic system and the pathophysiology of OMD involving impairments in proprioceptive pathways.

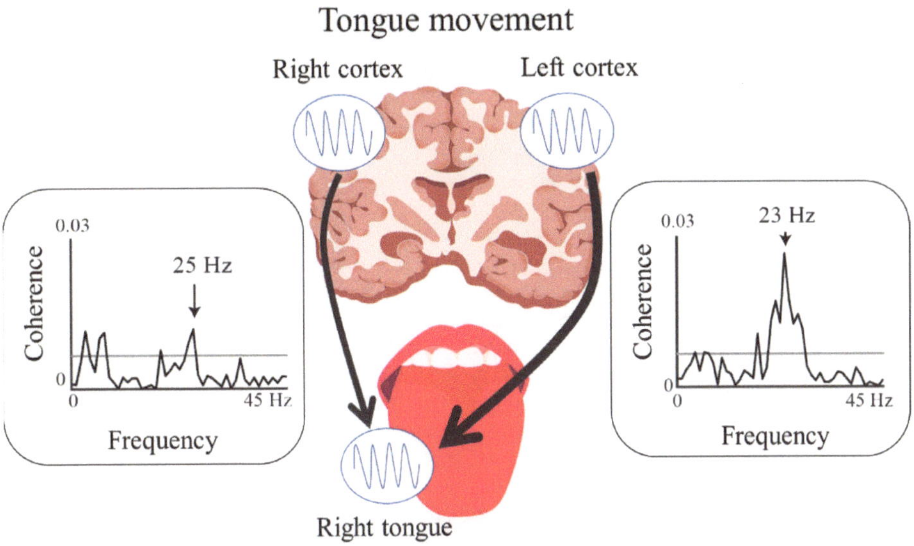

Figure 2. Bilateral functional connections between the cortex and tongue identified using corticomuscular coherence analysis. The figure shows contralateral (left hemispheric) dominance of the functional connection between the cortex and right side of the tongue.

3.3. Somatosensory-Evoked Fields and Potentials

Since the first reports of SEFs induced by trigeminal nerve stimulation in the early 1980s [44] and 1990s [45], many MEG studies have sought to assess SEF characteristics in the tongue [45–48], lips [49,50], palate [51,52], teeth [44], gingiva [49], and lower face [53].

Following tongue stimulation, the initial SEF components occur over the bilateral hemispheres at 19 ms with electrical stimulation [47] and 15 ms with tactile stimulation [48], with an anterior current orientation. These timings are consistent with a SEP latency of 16 ms following electrical stimulation of the lip via chronically implanted subdural electrodes over the lower perirolandic area in patients undergoing epilepsy surgery [54]. However, the initial component of trigeminal SEF/SEP is not detected stably due to the low amplitude of this component and is easily masked by excessive stimulation artefacts. Thus, in clinical settings, a prominent component with a large amplitude at a middle latency ranging from 25 ms to 80 ms, with a posterior current orientation, is often adopted [45,46,49,52,53,55]. Indeed, Previous studies reported that the middle-latency component of the trigeminal SEF can be used to evaluate sensory disturbances of the tongue and lip caused by injury to the trigeminal nerve during dental surgery [50,56,57]. Source localization studies involving MEG with high spatial resolution have revealed that the initial and middle-latency components of SEFs stimulated in the stomatognathic system are derived from the bilateral S1, specifically, the posterior bank of the central sulcus [46–50]. This neurophysiological finding is consistent with the anatomical principle that the unilateral lingual nerve innervating the anterior part of the tongue projects to both sides of area 3b in S1 via the trigeminothalamic tract, with contralateral dominance.

4. Oromandibular Dystonia

4.1. Pathophysiology of OMD

Although the pathogenesis of primary dystonia is still a matter of debate, several probable explanations have been proposed, including basal ganglia dysfunction, hyperexcitability of motor neurons, loss of inhibition, aberrant dopamine signaling, monoaminergic dysfunction, abnormal plasticity, and abnormal sensory function [58–61]. Most previous EEG studies of focal dystonia in humans have focused on cortical sensorimotor dysfunction, especially of the primary sensorimotor cortex and premotor areas, in cases affecting the hand (e.g., writer's cramp) [59].

MRCPs associated with hand movements consisted of at least two slow negative shifts. The early component is the BP, which is maximal at the vertex and symmetrically distributed over the scalp, whereas the latter component is called NS′, which is largest in the central area contralateral to the hand movement [62]. The BP represents the activation of supplementary motor areas (SMAs), while NS′ reflects activities in both the SMA and M1 [63–65]. However, the precise anatomical representations of the BP and NS′ remain controversial.

Several EEG studies have reported abnormalities in MRCPs in patients with focal dystonia [66–68]. Reductions in both NS′ and BP gradients have been observed in patients with symptomatic dystonia caused by lesions in the basal ganglia and anterior thalamus. Furthermore, reductions in NS′ amplitude over the contralateral central region have been observed in patients with writer's cramp [66,67]. These results suggest impaired activation of the sensorimotor cortex contralateral to the affected hand immediately before a voluntary movement. One study also reported abnormalities in the cortical preparatory processes for voluntary muscle relaxation or motor inhibition in patients with focal hand dystonia [68]. The BP associated with voluntary muscle relaxation was reduced over the central region of the affected hemisphere in patients with focal hand dystonia, suggesting impaired activation of the inhibitory motor systems in the contralateral cortex in these patients [68]. Moreover, a functional magnetic resonance imaging (fMRI) study reported smaller activation volumes in the SMA proper and primary sensorimotor cortex during voluntary muscle contraction and relaxation of the affected (right) hand in patients with writer's cramp than in healthy volunteers [69]. Disturbances in sensorimotor integration have also been documented as a task-specific decrease in the amplitude of contingent negative variation [70,71], abnormal pre-movement gating of somatosensory input [72], and abnormal CMC with MEG [73]. Other studies using paired-pulse transcranial magnetic stimulation have reported impairments in short-interval intracortical inhibition [74] and surround inhibition [75]. Somatotopic disorganization of the fingers has also been observed in the S1 contralateral to the affected hand [76]. These findings collectively demonstrate that focal dystonia of the hand involves impaired cortical inhibition in M1, abnormal sensorimotor integration, and disorganization of S1 [69,70].

A few EEG studies have also investigated the pathological characteristics of OMD. A study compared MRCPs associated with mandibular movements in six patients with OMD and eight healthy controls [35]. In the patient group, MRCP amplitudes over the central and parietal areas for mouth opening and lateral movements were significantly reduced compared to those observed in the control group. Moreover, in controls, the MRCPs at mouth opening and closing were symmetrically distributed, whereas those at lateral movements were predominant over the hemisphere ipsilateral to the direction of movement. This laterality was lost in the patient group. These results suggest that OMD is associated with bilateral impairments in cortical preparatory processing during jaw movement. A few studies have also investigated OMD pathology using fMRI and positron emission tomography. One fMRI study reported reduced activation of the primary sensorimotor cortex and premotor/sensory association cortices during vocalization in patients with laryngeal dystonia [77]. Analogous to the motor dysfunction observed in patients with dystonia, reduced primary somatosensory activity has previously been demonstrated [78,79], supporting the conceptualization of dystonia as a partial sensory disorder [80,81].

4.2. Treatment Options for OMD

BoNT injection represents the standard therapy for patients with focal dystonia such as blepharospasm, cervical dystonia, and OMD [82–84]. When the target muscles, doses, and patient expectations are appropriately managed, BoNT injection is a safe and effective approach for the treatment of OMD [3]. Some studies reported the effectiveness of ultrasound-guided injections in facial muscles to avoid injuring the neural vascular structures during botulinum toxin injection [85,86].

BoNT is a microbial protein that exists in seven serotypes, designated A through G. Its ability to block acetylcholine release at the NMJ accounts for its therapeutic effects in various movement disorders associated with increased muscle tone or muscle overactivity. BoNT wields these effects by entering nerve endings at the NMJ and cleaving soluble N-ethylmaleimide-sensitive factor-attachment protein receptors, thereby preventing the vesicular release of acetylcholine from the synaptic terminal and producing the effects of muscle relaxation and flaccid paralysis [87,88].

In addition to the effect on the peripheral nervous system, BoNT may also indirectly influence the functional organization of the central nervous system associated with altered peripheral inputs [89,90]. Moreover, the central effect of BoNT injection is not limited to the cortical and subcortical regions of the treated muscles but extends beyond the neural circuits for the control of the affected body parts [89,91,92]. Further studies with non-invasive brain-imaging techniques, including MEG and EEG, may help to reveal the bilateral cortical areas affected by therapy with BoNT injection in patients with OMD.

Other treatments for focal dystonia include invasive approaches, such as DBS, targeting central regions [93–95]. When symptoms cannot be adequately managed through medication and rehabilitation, DBS is typically employed as a surgical intervention to treat movement disorders. The main DBS target for dystonia treatment is the internal segment of the GPi [96], which has proven efficacious in the treatment of generalized, segmental, and cervical dystonia [97–99]. Although evidence concerning the efficacy of DBS for other dystonia subtypes remains scarce, DBS targeting the GPi has demonstrated continued efficacy in patients with Meige syndrome [94,100–102]. A recent meta-analysis showed that DBS may be useful for treating refractory Meige syndrome [103]. However, other studies have demonstrated that in some patients with craniocervical and craniofacial segmental dystonia, DBS is ineffective for improving stomatognathic functions such as speech and swallowing but is effective for improving blepharospasm [95,104,105]. A recent study of DBS in 18 patients with dystonia related to *KMT2B* mutations reported that the greatest improvements in motor function were observed in patients with trunk and cervical dystonia, with less clinical impact observed in patients with laryngeal dystonia [106].

Currently, only three published case reports have discussed bilateral GPi-DBS for OMD, all of which were categorized as lingual dystonia. Chung et al. [20] and Asahi et al. [22] reported symptomatic improvements in lingual dystonia following bilateral GPi-DBS in two cases and one case, respectively. In patients with OMD, the unique neuroanatomical characteristics of bilateral innervation in each side of the stomatognathic system may complicate the application of conventional DBS compared to that in patients with focal dystonia of the limbs, as previous studies have reported that sufficient effects are sometimes difficult to obtain with interventions targeting the unilateral hemisphere. As contralateral dominance is involved in the control of voluntary movement in the stomatognathic system, it may be beneficial for future research to explore the most effective stimulation parameters for bilateral DBS targeting the GPi in patients with OMD. However, some patients' OMD symptoms do not improve sufficiently even after DBS, and they require additional BoNT therapy. A highly individualized injection technique has been developed for lingual dystonia according to the direction of deviation [107]. An improved understanding of the central and peripheral mechanisms related to stomatognathic functions may promote the development of new treatments for OMD, such as the combination of BoNT injection into the affected muscles as peripheral therapy and DBS as central therapy.

Several authors have also discussed the use of unique oral appliances (e.g., oral splints) for OMD treatment [108–113]. Previous research has shown that performing certain sensory tricks (e.g., pressing the teeth or lips with the fingers; placing cigarettes, chewing gum, or other objects in the mouth; singing; and humming) may benefit a third of patients with OMD [109,114,115]. Oral appliances may be particularly useful in cases where they successfully mimic the patient's sensory tricks [109,114], as treatment responses in such patients may be linked to sensory tricks perceived by the brain to be beneficial. Although the precise mechanism underlying this phenomenon remains unknown, the beneficial effect of splint use on OMD may be related to the modulation of hyperactive dystonic networks by altered proprioceptive feedback and antagonist activation [114]. MEG recordings with CKC and low-CMC analyses are useful for evaluating proprioceptive feedback from muscles to the cortex during voluntary movements in the stomatognathic system (see Section 3.2). These approaches may aid in revealing the effects of oral appliance therapy on abnormal cortical activity related to proprioceptive feedback in patients with OMD.

5. Future Directions

BoNT injection is the standard peripheral therapy for patients with OMD. In addition, central therapies such as bilateral DBS can be applied, providing substantial relief in patients with disordered movements. However, the introduction of stimulating electrodes deep in the brain carries significant risks, including the risk of hemorrhage [116]. Beyond DBS, recent studies have highlighted the potential of non-invasive cortical current stimulation therapies such as transcranial direct current stimulation (tDCS) [117,118] and transcranial alternating-current stimulation (tACS) [119] for patients with limb movement disorders, although their effectiveness and mechanisms of action are still unclear [120–122]. For example, a previous study successfully reported the non-invasive application of tACS over the M1 [119], which induced phase cancellation of the resting tremor rhythm in the upper limbs of healthy volunteers. In the future, applying tACS over the bilateral M1 in the stomatognathic system may aid in the treatment of OMD given the bilateral cortical control of this system. Indeed, in our previous study, tDCS of the bilateral M1 area representing the tongue region significantly increased the excitability of this region and improved tongue motor functions compared to the application of tDCS to the unilateral M1 of the tongue region in healthy volunteers [123].

6. Conclusions

In this review, we provide an overview of the unique central spatiotemporal processing mechanisms in the stomatognathic system. The uncertain effects of DBS on OMD may, in part, be explained by the unique characteristics of the bilateral central regulation of sensorimotor functions in the stomatognathic system. Further exploration of the neurophysiological underpinnings of stomatognathic functions will lead to an improved understanding of the etiology of OMD and may lead to innovative approaches for future symptomatic and disease-modifying treatments.

7. Methods

This literature review was conducted based on the comprehensive analysis of electronic medical literature databases (PubMed, Scopus, EMBASE, and Google scholar) prior to 1 September 2022. Search keywords included oromandibular dystonia, orofacial dystonia, mandibular dystonia, jaw dystonia, lingual dystonia, Meige syndrome, botulinum toxin, botulinum toxin therapy, deep brain stimulation, transcranial direct current stimulation (tDCS), and transcranial alternating-current stimulation (tACS) for Sections 1, 4 and 5 of the manuscript. We also searched the terms trigeminal nerve, lingual nerve, tongue, palate, face, lip, oromandibular, stomatognathic system, sensory disturbance, sensory abnormality, electroencephalography (EEG), and magnetoencephalography (MEG) for Sections 1–3 and Section 5. Each search result was independently reviewed for eligibility by the author (H.M.). No restriction was placed with respect to the original text language.

Author Contributions: Conceptualization, H.M. and K.Y.; Writing–Original Draft Preparation, H.M.; Writing–Review and Editing, K.Y. and M.H.; Funding Acquisition, H.M. All authors have read and agreed to the published version of the manuscript.

Funding: This research was funded by JSPS KAKENHI, grant numbers JP19K10218 and JP22H03452 to H.M.

Institutional Review Board Statement: Not applicable.

Informed Consent Statement: Not applicable.

Data Availability Statement: Not applicable.

Conflicts of Interest: The authors declare no conflict of interest.

References

1. Comella, C.L. Systematic review of botulinum toxin treatment for oromandibular dystonia. *Toxicon* **2018**, *147*, 96–99. [CrossRef] [PubMed]
2. Scorr, L.M.; Factor, S.A.; Parra, S.P.; Kaye, R.; Paniello, R.C.; Norris, S.A.; Perlmutter, J.S.; Bäumer, T.; Usnich, T.; Berman, B.D.; et al. Oromandibular dystonia: A clinical examination of 2020 cases. *Front. Neurol.* **2021**, *12*, 700714. [CrossRef]
3. Yoshida, K. Botulinum toxin therapy for oromandibular dystonia and other movement disorders in the stomatognathic system. *Toxins* **2022**, *14*, 282. [CrossRef] [PubMed]
4. Albanese, A.; Bhatia, K.; Bressman, S.B.; Delong, M.R.; Fahn, S.; Fung, V.S.; Hallett, M.; Jankovic, J.; Jinnah, H.A.; Klein, C.; et al. Phenomenology and classification of dystonia: A consensus update. *Mov. Disord.* **2013**, *28*, 863–873. [CrossRef] [PubMed]
5. Colosimo, C.; Berardelli, A. Clinical phenomenology of dystonia. *Int. Rev. Neurobiol.* **2011**, *98*, 509–524. [CrossRef] [PubMed]
6. Manzo, N.; Ginatempo, F.; Belvisi, D.; Defazio, G.; Conte, A.; Deriu, F.; Berardelli, A. Pathophysiological mechanisms of oromandibular dystonia. *Clin. Neurophysiol.* **2022**, *134*, 73–80. [CrossRef] [PubMed]
7. Yoshida, K. Development and validation of a disease-specific oromandibular dystonia rating scale (OMDRS). *Front. Neurol.* **2020**, *11*, 583177. [CrossRef]
8. Meige, H. Les convulsions de la face: Une forme clinique de convulsion faciale, bilatérale et médiane. *Rev. Neurol.* **1910**, *10*, 437–443.
9. Weiss, E.M.; Hershey, T.; Karimi, M.; Racette, B.; Tabbal, S.D.; Mink, J.W.; Paniello, R.C.; Perlmutter, J.S. Relative risk of spread of symptoms among the focal onset primary dystonias. *Mov. Disord.* **2006**, *21*, 1175–1181. [CrossRef]
10. Abbruzzese, G.; Berardelli, A.; Girlanda, P.; Marchese, R.; Martino, D.; Morgante, F.; Avanzino, L.; Colosimo, C.; Defazio, G. Long-term assessment of the risk of spread in primary late-onset focal dystonia. *J. Neurol. Neurosurg. Psychiatry* **2008**, *79*, 392–396. [CrossRef]
11. Pandey, S.; Sharma, S. Meige's syndrome: History, epidemiology, clinical features, pathogenesis and treatment. *J. Neurol. Sci.* **2017**, *15*, 162–170. [CrossRef] [PubMed]
12. Pirio Richardson, S.; Wegele, A.R.; Skipper, B.; Deligtisch, A.; Jinnah, H.A.; Dystonia Coalition Investigators. Dystonia treatment: Patterns of medication use in an international cohort. *Neurology* **2017**, *88*, 543–550. [CrossRef] [PubMed]
13. Steeves, T.D.; Day, L.; Dykeman, J.; Jette, N.; Pringsheim, T. The prevalence of primary dystonia: A systematic review and meta-analysis. *Mov. Disord.* **2012**, *27*, 1789–1796. [CrossRef] [PubMed]
14. Nutt, J.G.; Muenter, M.D.; Aronson, A.; Kurland, L.T.; Melton, L.J. Epidemiology of focal and generalized dystonia in Rochester, Minnesota. *Mov. Disord.* **1988**, *3*, 188–194. [CrossRef]
15. Cardoso, F.; Jankovic, J. Dystonia and dyskinesia. *Psychiatr. Clin. N. Am.* **1997**, *20*, 821–838. [CrossRef]
16. Yoshida, K. Prevalence and incidence of oromandibular dystonia: An oral and maxillofacial surgery service-based study. *Clin. Oral Investig.* **2021**, *25*, 5755–5764. [CrossRef]
17. Hallett, M.; Benecke, R.; Blitzer, A.; Comella, C.L. Treatment of focal dystonias with botulinum neurotoxin. *Toxicon* **2009**, *54*, 628–633. [CrossRef]
18. Tisch, S. Deep brain stimulation in dystonia: Factors contributing to variability in outcome in short and long term follow-up. *Curr. Opin. Neurol.* **2022**, *35*, 510–517. [CrossRef]
19. Schneider, S.A.; Aggarwal, A.; Bhatt, M.; Dupont, E.; Tisch, S.; Limousin, P.; Lee, P.; Quinn, N.; Bhatia, K.P. Severe tongue protrusion dystonia: Clinical syndromes and possible treatment. *Neurology* **2006**, *67*, 940–943. [CrossRef]
20. Chung, J.C.; Kim, J.P.; Chang, W.S.; Kim, H.Y.; Chang, J.W. Bilateral pallidal stimulation for "sticking-out tongue" feature in patients with primary focal tongue protrusion dystonia. *Neuromodulation* **2014**, *17*, 133–137. [CrossRef]
21. Wu, Y.; Pan, Y.; Huang, P.; Wang, T.; Zhang, C.; Sun, B.; Li, D.; Li, H.; Wu, Y. Subthalamic deep brain stimulation in lingual dystonia: A case series study. *Park. Relat. Disord.* **2021**, *88*, 114–115. [CrossRef] [PubMed]
22. Asahi, T.; Ikeda, K.; Yamamoto, J.; Tsubono, H.; Muro, Y.; Sato, S. Bilateral pallidal stimulation with directional leads for primary focal lingual dystonia. *Stereotact. Funct. Neurosurg.* **2021**, *99*, 207–211. [CrossRef]
23. Hari, R.; Salmelin, R. Magnetoencephalography: From SQUIDs to neuroscience. Neuroimage 20th anniversary special edition. *Neuroimage* **2012**, *61*, 386–396. [CrossRef] [PubMed]

24. Penfield, W.; Boldrey, E. Somatic motor and sensory representation in the cerebral cortex of man as studied by electrical stimulation. *Brain* **1937**, *60*, 389–443. [CrossRef]
25. Kubota, K.; Masegi, T. Muscle spindle supply to the human jaw muscle. *J. Dent. Res.* **1977**, *56*, 901–909. [CrossRef] [PubMed]
26. Nakamura, A.; Yamada, T.; Goto, A.; Kato, T.; Ito, K.; Abe, Y.; Kachi, T.; Kakigi, R. Somatosensory homunculus as drawn by MEG. *Neuroimage* **1998**, *7*, 377–386. [CrossRef]
27. Deecke, L.; Weinberg, H.; Brickett, P. Magnetic fields of the human brain accompanying voluntary movement: Bereitschaftsmagnetfeld. *Exp. Brain Res.* **1982**, *48*, 144–148. [CrossRef]
28. Hari, R.; Antervo, A.; Katila, T.; Poutanen, T.; Seppänen, M.; Tuomisto, T.; Varpula, T. Cerebral magnetic fields associated with voluntary limb movements in man. *Il Nuovo Cimento D* **1983**, *2*, 484–494. [CrossRef]
29. Cheyne, D.; Kristeva, R.; Deecke, L. Homuncular organization of human motor cortex as indicated by neuromagnetic recordings. *Neurosci. Lett.* **1991**, *122*, 17–20. [CrossRef]
30. Nakasato, N.; Itoh, H.; Hatanaka, K.; Nakahara, H.; Kanno, A.; Yoshimoto, T. Movement-related magnetic fields to tongue protrusion. *Neuroimage* **2001**, *14*, 924–935. [CrossRef]
31. Maezawa, H.; Oguma, H.; Hirai, Y.; Hisadome, K.; Shiraishi, H.; Funahashi, M. Movement-related cortical magnetic fields associated with self-paced tongue protrusion in humans. *Neurosci. Res.* **2017**, *117*, 22–27. [CrossRef] [PubMed]
32. Nagamine, T.; Kajola, M.; Salmelin, R.; Shibasaki, H.; Hari, R. Movement-related slow cortical magnetic fields and changes of spontaneous MEG- and EEG-brain rhythms. *Electroencephalogr. Clin. Neurophysiol.* **1996**, *99*, 274–286. [CrossRef]
33. Kornhuber, H.H.; Deecke, L. Changes in the brain potential in voluntary movements and passive movements in man: Readiness potential and reafferent potentials. *Pflüger's Arch. Gesamte Physiol. Menschen Tiere* **1965**, *284*, 1–17. [CrossRef]
34. Yoshida, K.; Kaji, R.; Hamano, T.; Kohara, N.; Kimura, J.; Shibasaki, H.; Iizuka, T. Cortical potentials associated with voluntary mandibular movements. *J. Dent. Res.* **2000**, *79*, 1514–1518. [CrossRef] [PubMed]
35. Yoshida, K.; Kaji, R.; Kohara, N.; Murase, N.; Ikeda, A.; Shibasaki, H.; Iizuka, T. Movement-related cortical potentials before jaw excursions in oromandibular dystonia. *Mov. Disord.* **2003**, *18*, 94–100. [CrossRef]
36. Shibukawa, Y.; Shintani, M.; Kumai, T.; Suzuki, T.; Nakamura, Y. Cortical neuromagnetic fields preceding voluntary jaw movements. *J. Dent. Res.* **2004**, *83*, 572–577. [CrossRef]
37. Conway, B.A.; Halliday, D.M.; Farmer, S.F.; Shahani, U.; Maas, P.; Weir, A.I.; Rosenberg, J.R. Synchronization between motor cortex and spinal motoneuronal pool during the performance of a maintained motor task in man. *J. Physiol.* **1995**, *489*, 917–924. [CrossRef]
38. Mima, T.; Hallett, M. Corticomuscular coherence: A review. *J. Clin. Neurophysiol.* **1999**, *16*, 501–511. [CrossRef]
39. Maezawa, H.; Mima, T.; Yazawa, S.; Matsuhashi, M.; Shiraishi, H.; Hirai, Y.; Funahashi, M. Contralateral dominance of corticomuscular coherence for both sides of the tongue during human tongue protrusion: An MEG study. *Neuroimage* **2014**, *101*, 245–255. [CrossRef]
40. Maezawa, H.; Mima, T.; Yazawa, S.; Matsuhashi, M.; Shiraishi, H.; Funahashi, M. Cortico-muscular synchronization by proprioceptive afferents from the tongue muscles during isometric tongue protrusion. *Neuroimage* **2016**, *128*, 284–292. [CrossRef]
41. Bourguignon, M.; De Tiège, X.; Op de Beeck, M.; Pirotte, B.; Van Bogaert, P.; Goldman, S.; Hari, R.; Jousmäki, V. Functional motor-cortex mapping using corticokinematic coherence. *Neuroimage* **2011**, *55*, 1475–1479. [CrossRef] [PubMed]
42. Bourguignon, M.; Piitulainen, H.; De Tiège, X.; Jousmäki, V.; Hari, R. Corticokinematic coherence mainly reflects movement-induced proprioceptive feedback. *Neuroimage* **2015**, *106*, 382–390. [CrossRef]
43. Maezawa, H.; Fujimoto, M.; Hata, Y.; Matsuhashi, M.; Hashimoto, H.; Kashioka, H.; Yanagida, T.; Hirata, M. Functional cortical localization of tongue movements using corticokinematic coherence with a deep learning-assisted motion capture system. *Sci. Rep.* **2022**, *12*, 388. [CrossRef] [PubMed]
44. Hari, R.; Kaukoranta, E.; Reinikainen, K.; Huopaniemie, T.; Mauno, J. Neuromagnetic localization of cortical activity evoked by painful dental stimulation in man. *Neurosci. Lett.* **1983**, *42*, 77–82. [CrossRef]
45. Karhu, J.; Hari, R.; Lu, S.T.; Paetau, R.; Rif, J. Cerebral magnetic fields to lingual stimulation. *Electroencephalogr. Clin. Neurophysiol.* **1991**, *80*, 459–468. [CrossRef]
46. Maezawa, H.; Yoshida, K.; Nagamine, T.; Matsubayashi, J.; Enatsu, R.; Bessho, K.; Fukuyama, H. Somatosensory evoked magnetic fields following electric tongue stimulation using pin electrodes. *Neurosci. Res.* **2008**, *62*, 131–139. [CrossRef]
47. Sakamoto, K.; Nakata, H.; Kakigi, R. Somatosensory-evoked magnetic fields following stimulation of the tongue in humans. *Clin. Neurophysiol.* **2008**, *119*, 1664–1673. [CrossRef]
48. Tamura, Y.; Shibukawa, Y.; Shintani, M.; Kaneko, Y.; Ichinohe, T. Oral structure representation in human somatosensory cortex. *Neuroimage* **2008**, *43*, 128–135. [CrossRef]
49. Nakahara, H.; Nakasato, N.; Kanno, A.; Murayama, S.; Hatanaka, K.; Itoh, H.; Yoshimoto, T. Somatosensory-evoked fields for gingiva, lip, and tongue. *J. Dent. Res.* **2004**, *83*, 307–311. [CrossRef]
50. Maezawa, H.; Matsuhashi, M.; Yoshida, K.; Mima, T.; Nagamine, T.; Fukuyama, H. Evaluation of lip sensory disturbance using somatosensory evoked magnetic fields. *Clin. Neurophysiol.* **2014**, *125*, 363–369. [CrossRef]
51. Yoshida, K.; Maezawa, H.; Nagamine, T.; Fukuyama, H.; Murakami, K.; Iizuka, T. Somatosensory evoked magnetic fields to air-puff stimulation on the soft palate. *Neurosci. Res.* **2006**, *55*, 116–122. [CrossRef] [PubMed]
52. Maezawa, H.; Hirai, Y.; Shiraishi, H.; Funahashi, M. Somatosensory evoked magnetic fields following tongue and hard palate stimulation on the preferred chewing side. *J. Neurol. Sci.* **2014**, *347*, 288–294. [CrossRef] [PubMed]

53. Yamashita, H.; Kumamoto, Y.; Nakashima, T.; Yamamoto, T.; Inokuchi, A.; Komiyama, S. Magnetic sensory cortical responses evoked by tactile stimulations of the human face, oral cavity and flap reconstructions of the tongue. *Eur. Arch. Otorhinolaryngol.* **1999**, *256* (Suppl. S1), S42–S46. [CrossRef] [PubMed]
54. Ikeda, A.; Lüders, H.O.; Burgess, R.C.; Sakamoto, A.; Klem, G.H.; Morris, H.H.; Shibasaki, H. Generator locations of movement-related potentials with tongue protrusions and vocalizations: Subdural recording in human. *Electroencephalogr. Clin. Neurophysiol.* **1995**, *96*, 310–328. [CrossRef]
55. Disbrow, E.A.; Hinkley, L.B.; Roberts, T.P. Ipsilateral representation of oral structures in human anterior parietal somatosensory cortex and integration of inputs across the midline. *J. Comp. Neurol.* **2003**, *467*, 487–495. [CrossRef] [PubMed]
56. Maezawa, H.; Yoshida, K.; Matsuhashi, M.; Yokoyama, Y.; Mima, T.; Bessho, K.; Fujita, S.; Nagamine, T.; Fukuyama, H. Evaluation of tongue sensory disturbance by somatosensory evoked magnetic fields following tongue stimulation. *Neurosci. Res.* **2011**, *71*, 244–250. [CrossRef]
57. Maezawa, H.; Tojyo, I.; Yoshida, K.; Fujita, S. Recovery of impaired somatosensory evoked fields after improvement of tongue sensory deficits with neurosurgical reconstruction. *J. Oral Maxillofac. Surg.* **2016**, *74*, 1473–1482. [CrossRef]
58. Hallett, M.; Kanchana, S. Pathophysiology of dystonia. In *Clinical Diagnosis and Management of Dystonia*; CRC Press: Abingdon, UK, 2007; pp. 43–51.
59. Vidailhet, M.; Grabli, D.; Roze, E. Pathophysiology of dystonia. *Curr. Opin. Neurol.* **2009**, *22*, 406–413. [CrossRef]
60. Skogseid, I.M. Dystonia—New advances in classification, genetics, pathophysiology and treatment. *Acta Neurol. Scand. Suppl.* **2014**, *198*, 13–19. [CrossRef]
61. Brüggemann, N. Contemporary functional neuroanatomy and pathophysiology of dystonia. *J. Neural Transm.* **2021**, *128*, 499–508. [CrossRef]
62. Shibasaki, H.; Hallett, M. What is the Bereitschaftspotential? *Clin. Neurophysiol.* **2006**, *117*, 2341–2356. [CrossRef] [PubMed]
63. Neshige, R.; Lüders, H.; Shibasaki, H. Recording of movement-related potentials from scalp and cortex in man. *Brain* **1988**, *111*, 719–736. [CrossRef] [PubMed]
64. Ikeda, A.; Lüders, H.O.; Burgess, R.C.; Shibasaki, H. Movement-related potentials recorded from supplementary motor area and primary motor area. Role of supplementary motor area in voluntary movements. *Brain* **1992**, *115*, 1017–1043. [CrossRef] [PubMed]
65. Shibasaki, H.; Sadato, N.; Lyshkow, H.; Yonekura, Y.; Honda, M.; Nagamine, T.; Suwazono, S.; Magata, Y.; Ikeda, A.; Miyazaki, M. Both primary motor cortex and supplementary motor area play an important role in complex finger movement. *Brain* **1993**, *116*, 1387–1398. [CrossRef]
66. Fève, A.; Bathien, N.; Rondot, P. Abnormal movement related potentials in patients with lesions of basal ganglia and anterior thalamus. *J. Neurol. Neurosurg. Psychiatry* **1994**, *57*, 100–104. [CrossRef]
67. Deuschl, G.; Toro, C.; Matsumoto, J.; Hallett, M. Movement-related cortical potentials in writer's cramp. *Ann. Neurol.* **1995**, *38*, 862–868. [CrossRef]
68. Yazawa, S.; Ikeda, A.; Kaji, R.; Terada, K.; Nagamine, T.; Toma, K.; Kubori, T.; Kimura, J.; Shibasaki, H. Abnormal cortical processing of voluntary muscle relaxation in patients with focal hand dystonia studied by movement-related potentials. *Brain* **1999**, *122*, 1357–1366. [CrossRef]
69. Oga, T.; Honda, M.; Toma, K.; Murase, N.; Okada, T.; Hanakawa, T.; Sawamoto, N.; Nagamine, T.; Konishi, J.; Fukuyama, H.; et al. Abnormal cortical mechanisms of voluntary muscle relaxation in patients with writer's cramp: An fMRI study. *Brain* **2002**, *125*, 895–903. [CrossRef]
70. Kaji, R.; Ikeda, A.; Ikeda, T.; Kubori, T.; Mezaki, T.; Kohara, N.; Kanda, M.; Nagamine, T.; Honda, M.; Rothwell, J.C. Physiological study of cervical dystonia. Task-specific abnormality in contingent negative variation. *Brain* **1995**, *118*, 511–522. [CrossRef]
71. Ikeda, A.; Shibasaki, H.; Kaji, R.; Terada, K.; Nagamine, T.; Honda, M.; Hamano, T.; Kimura, J. Abnormal sensorimotor integration in writer's cramp: Study of contingent negative variation. *Mov. Disord.* **1996**, *11*, 683–690. [CrossRef]
72. Murase, N.; Kaji, R.; Shimazu, H.; Katayama-Hirota, M.; Ikeda, A.; Kohara, N.; Kimura, J.; Shibasaki, H.; Rothwell, J.C. Abnormal premovement gating of somatosensory input in writer's cramp. *Brain* **2000**, *123*, 1813–1829. [CrossRef] [PubMed]
73. Tecchio, F.; Melgari, J.M.; Zappasodi, F.; Porcaro, C.; Milazzo, D.; Cassetta, E.; Rossini, P.M. Sensorimotor integration in focal task-specific hand dystonia: A magnetoencephalographic assessment. *Neuroscience* **2008**, *154*, 563–571. [CrossRef] [PubMed]
74. Ridding, M.C.; Sheean, G.; Rothwell, J.C.; Inzelberg, R.; Kujirai, T. Changes in the balance between motor cortical excitation and inhibition in focal, task specific dystonia. *J. Neurol. Neurosurg. Psychiatry.* **1995**, *59*, 493–498. [CrossRef] [PubMed]
75. Sohn, Y.H.; Hallett, M. Disturbed surround inhibition in focal hand dystonia. *Ann. Neurol.* **2004**, *56*, 595–599. [CrossRef]
76. Münte, T.F.; Altenmüller, E.; Jäncke, L. The musician's brain as a model of neuroplasticity. *Nat. Rev. Neurosci.* **2002**, *3*, 473–478. [CrossRef]
77. Haslinger, B.; Erhard, P.; Dresel, C.; Castrop, F.; Roettinger, M.; Ceballos-Baumann, A.O. 'Silent event-related' fMRI reveals reduced sensorimotor activation in laryngeal dystonia. *Neurology* **2005**, *65*, 1562–1569. [CrossRef]
78. Ceballos-Baumann, A.O.; Passingham, R.E.; Warner, T.; Playford, E.D.; Marsden, C.D.; Brooks, D.J. Overactive prefrontal and underactive motor cortical areas in idiopathic dystonia. *Ann. Neurol.* **1995**, *37*, 363–372. [CrossRef]
79. Tempel, L.W.; Perlmutter, J.S. Abnormal vibration-induced cerebral blood flow responses in idiopathic dystonia. *Brain* **1990**, *113*, 691–707. [CrossRef]

80. Tinazzi, M.; Rosso, T.; Fiaschi, A. Role of the somatosensory system in primary dystonia. *Mov. Disord.* **2003**, *18*, 605–622. [CrossRef]
81. Hallett, M. Is dystonia a sensory disorder? *Ann. Neurol.* **1995**, *38*, 139–140. [CrossRef]
82. Simpson, D.M.; Blitzer, A.; Brashear, A.; Comella, C.; Dubinsky, R.; Hallett, M.; Jankovic, J.; Karp, B.; Ludlow, C.L.; Miyasaki, J.M.; et al. Assessment: Botulinum neurotoxin for the treatment of movement disorders (an evidence-based review): Report of the Therapeutics and Technology Assessment Subcommittee of the American Academy of Neurology. *Neurology* **2008**, *70*, 1699–1706. [CrossRef] [PubMed]
83. Jankovic, J. An update on new and unique uses of botulinum toxin in movement disorders. *Toxicon* **2018**, *147*, 84–88. [CrossRef] [PubMed]
84. Anandan, C.; Jankovic, J. Botulinum toxin in movement disorders: An update. *Toxins* **2021**, *13*, 42. [CrossRef] [PubMed]
85. Lee, H.J.; Kim, J.S.; Youn, K.H.; Lee, J.; Kim, H.-J. Ultrasound-guided botulinum neurotoxin type A injection for correcting asymmetrical smiles. *Aesthet. Surg. J.* **2018**, *38*, 130–134. [CrossRef] [PubMed]
86. Wu, W.T.; Chang, K.V.; Chang, H.C.; Chen, L.R.; Kuan, C.H.; Kao, J.T.; Wei, L.Y.; Chen, Y.J.; Han, D.S.; Özçakar, L. Ultrasound imaging of the facial muscles and relevance with botulinum toxin injections: A pictorial essay and narrative review. *Toxins* **2022**, *27*, 101. [CrossRef]
87. Rossetto, O.; Pirazzini, M.; Montecucco, C. Botulinum neurotoxins: Genetic, structural and mechanistic insights. *Nat. Rev. Microbiol.* **2014**, *12*, 535549. [CrossRef]
88. Pirazzini, M.; Rossetto, O.; Eleopra, R.; Montecucco, C. Botulinum neurotoxins: Biology, pharmacology, and toxicology. *Pharmacol. Rev.* **2017**, *69*, 200235. [CrossRef]
89. Luvisetto, S. Botulinum neurotoxins in central nervous system: An overview from animal models to human therapy. *Toxins* **2021**, *13*, 751. [CrossRef]
90. Giladi, N. The mechanism of action of botulinum toxin type A in focal dystonia is most probably through its dual effect on efferent (motor) and afferent pathways at the injected site. *J. Neurol. Sci.* **1997**, *152*, 132135. [CrossRef]
91. Hok, P.; Veverka, T.; Hlustik, P.; Nevrly, M.; Kanovsky, P. The central effects of botulinum toxin in dystonia and spasticity. *Toxins* **2021**, *13*, 155. [CrossRef]
92. Weise, D.; Weise, C.M.; Naumann, M. Central effects of botulinum neurotoxin-Evidence from human studies. *Toxins* **2019**, *11*, 21. [CrossRef] [PubMed]
93. Ghang, J.Y.; Lee, M.K.; Jun, S.M.; Ghang, C.G. Outcome of pallidal deep brain stimulation in Meige syndrome. *J. Korean Neurosurg. Soc.* **2010**, *48*, 134–138. [CrossRef] [PubMed]
94. Lyons, M.K.; Birch, B.D.; Hillman, R.A.; Boucher, O.K.; Evidente, V.G. Long-term follow-up of deep brain stimulation for Meige syndrome. *Neurosurg. Focus* **2010**, *29*, E5. [CrossRef]
95. Ostrem, J.L.; Marks, W.J.; Volz, M.M.; Heath, S.L.; Starr, P.A. Pallidal deep brain stimulation in patients with cranial-cervical dystonia (Meige syndrome). *Mov. Disord.* **2007**, *22*, 1885–1891. [CrossRef] [PubMed]
96. Cury, R.G.; Kalia, S.K.; Shah, B.B.; Jimenez-Shahed, J.; Prashanth, L.K.; Moro, E. Surgical treatment of dystonia. *Expert Rev. Neurother.* **2018**, *18*, 477–492. [CrossRef] [PubMed]
97. Kupsch, A.; Benecke, R.; Müller, J.; Trottenberg, T.; Schneider, G.H.; Poewe, W.; Eisner, W.; Wolters, A.; Müller, J.U.; Deuschl, G.; et al. Pallidal deep-brain stimulation in primary generalized or segmental dystonia. *N. Engl. J. Med.* **2006**, *355*, 1978–1990. [CrossRef] [PubMed]
98. Albanese, A.; Asmus, F.; Bhatia, K.P.; Elia, A.E.; Elibol, B.; Filippini, G.; Gasser, T.; Krauss, J.K.; Nardocci, N.; Newton, A.; et al. EFNS guidelines on diagnosis and treatment of primary dystonias. *Eur. J. Neurol.* **2011**, *18*, 5–18. [CrossRef]
99. Tagliati, M.; Krack, P.; Volkmann, J.; Aziz, T.; Krauss, J.K.; Kupsch, A.; Vidailhet, A.M. Long-term management of DBS in dystonia: Response to stimulation, adverse events, battery changes, and special considerations. *Mov. Disord.* **2011**, *26* (Suppl. S1), S54–S62. [CrossRef]
100. Horisawa, S.; Ochiai, T.; Goto, S.; Nakajima, T.; Takeda, N.; Kawamata, T.; Taira, T. Long-term outcome of pallidal stimulation for Meige syndrome. *J. Neurosurg.* **2018**, *130*, 84–89. [CrossRef]
101. Sako, W.; Morigaki, R.; Mizobuchi, Y.; Tsuzuki, T.; Ima, H.; Ushio, Y.; Nagahiro, S.; Kaji, R.; Goto, S. Bilateral pallidal deep brain stimulation in primary Meige syndrome. *Parkinsonism Relat. Disord.* **2011**, *17*, 123–125. [CrossRef]
102. Inoue, N.; Nagahiro, S.; Kaji, R.; Goto, S. Long-term suppression of Meige syndrome after pallidal stimulation: A 10-year follow-up study. *Mov. Disord.* **2010**, *25*, 1756–1758. [CrossRef] [PubMed]
103. Wang, X.; Zhang, Z.; Mao, Z.; Yu, X. Deep brain stimulation for Meige syndrome: A meta-analysis with individual patient data. *J. Neurol.* **2019**, *266*, 2646–2656. [CrossRef]
104. Limotai, N.; Go, C.; Oyama, G.; Hwynn, N.; Zesiewicz, T.; Foote, K.; Bhidayasiri, R.; Malaty, I.; Zeilman, P.; Rodriguez, R.; et al. Mixed results for GPi-DBS in the treatment of cranio-facial and cranio-cervical dystonia symptoms. *J. Neurol.* **2011**, *258*, 2069–2074. [CrossRef] [PubMed]
105. Vidailhet, M.; Jutras, M.F.; Grabli, D.; Roze, E. Deep brain stimulation for dystonia. *J. Neurol. Neurosurg. Psychiatry* **2013**, *84*, 1029–1042. [CrossRef] [PubMed]
106. Cif, L.; Demailly, D.; Lin, J.P.; Barwick, K.E.; Sa, M.; Abela, L.; Malhotra, S.; Chong, W.K.; Steel, D.; Sanchis-Juan, A.; et al. KMT2B-related disorders: Expansion of the phenotypic spectrum and long-term efficacy of deep brain stimulation. *Brain* **2020**, *143*, 3242–3261. [CrossRef]

107. Yoshida, K. Botulinum neurotoxin therapy for lingual dystonia using an individualized injection method based on clinical features. *Toxins* **2019**, *11*, 51. [CrossRef]
108. Frucht, S.; Fahn, S.; Ford, B.; Gelb, M. A geste antagoniste device to treat jaw-closing dystonia. *Mov. Disord.* **1999**, *14*, 883–886. [CrossRef]
109. Lo, S.E.; Gelb, M.; Frucht, S.J. Geste antagonistes in idiopathic lower cranial dystonia. *Mov. Disord.* **2007**, *22*, 1012–1017. [CrossRef]
110. Satoh, M.; Narita, M.; Tomimoto, H. Three cases of focal embouchure dystonia: Classifications and successful therapy using a dental splint. *Eur. Neurol.* **2011**, *66*, 85–90. [CrossRef]
111. Yoshida, K. Sensory trick splint as a multimodal therapy for oromandibular dystonia. *J. Prosthodont. Res.* **2018**, *62*, 239–244. [CrossRef]
112. De Meyer, M.; Vereecke, L.; Bottenberg, P.; Jacquet, W.; Sims, A.B.; Santens, P. Oral appliances in the treatment of oromandibular dystonia: A systematic review. *Acta Neurol. Belg.* **2020**, *120*, 831–836. [CrossRef] [PubMed]
113. Gonzalez-Alegre, P.; Schneider, R.L.; Hoffman, H. Clinical, etiological, and therapeutic features of jaw-opening and jaw-closing oromandibular dystonias: A decade of experience at a single treatment center. *Tremor Other Hyperkinet. Mov.* **2014**, *4*, 231. [CrossRef]
114. Schramm, A.; Classen, J.; Reiners, K.; Naumann, M. Characteristics of sensory trick-like manoeuvres in jaw-opening dystonia. *Mov. Disord.* **2007**, *22*, 430–433. [CrossRef] [PubMed]
115. Sankhla, C.; Lai, E.C.; Jankovic, J. Peripherally induced oromandibular dystonia. *J. Neurol. Neurosurg. Psychiatry* **1998**, *65*, 722–728. [CrossRef] [PubMed]
116. Schiefer, T.K.; Matsumoto, J.Y.; Lee, K.H. Moving forward: Advances in the treatment of movement disorders with deep brain stimulation. *Front. Integr. Neurosci.* **2011**, *5*, 69. [CrossRef]
117. Marceglia, S.; Mrakic-Sposta, S.; Fumagalli, M.; Ferrucci, R.; Mameli, F.; Vergari, M.; Barbieri, S.; Priori, A. Cathodal transcranial direct current stimulation improves focal hand dystonia in musicians: A two-case study. *Front. Neurosci.* **2017**, *11*, 508. [CrossRef]
118. Young, S.J.; Bertucco, M.; Sheehan-Stross, R.; Sanger, T.D. Cathodal transcranial direct current stimulation in children with dystonia: A pilot open-label trial. *J. Child Neurol.* **2013**, *28*, 1238–1244. [CrossRef]
119. Brittain, J.S.; Probert-Smith, P.; Aziz, T.Z.; Brown, P. Tremor suppression by rhythmic transcranial current stimulation. *Curr. Biol.* **2013**, *23*, 436–440. [CrossRef]
120. Buttkus, F.; Weidenmüller, M.; Schneider, S.; Jabusch, H.C.; Nitsche, M.A.; Paulus, W.; Altenmüller, E. Failure of cathodal direct current stimulation to improve fine motor control in musician's dystonia. *Mov. Disord.* **2010**, *25*, 389–394. [CrossRef]
121. Benninger, D.H.; Lomarev, M.; Lopez, G.; Pal, N.; Luckenbaugh, D.A.; Hallett, M. Transcranial direct current stimulation for the treatment of focal hand dystonia. *Mov. Disord.* **2011**, *26*, 1698–1702. [CrossRef]
122. Bhanpuri, N.H.; Bertucco, M.; Young, S.J.; Lee, A.A.; Sanger, T.D. Multiday transcranial direct current stimulation causes clinically insignificant changes in childhood dystonia: A pilot study. *J. Child Neurol.* **2015**, *30*, 1604–1615. [CrossRef] [PubMed]
123. Maezawa, H.; Vicario, C.M.; Kuo, M.F.; Hirata, M.; Mima, T.; Nitsche, M.A. Effects of bilateral anodal transcranial direct current stimulation over the tongue primary motor cortex on cortical excitability of the tongue and tongue motor functions. *Brain Stimul.* **2020**, *13*, 270–272. [CrossRef] [PubMed]

toxins

Review

Botulinum Toxin, a Drug with Potential Interest for Dentists—An Introduction

Merete Bakke

Clinical Oral Physiology, Department of Odontology, Faculty of Health and Medical Sciences, University of Copenhagen, DK-2200 Copenhagen, Denmark; mbak@sund.ku.dk

Abstract: The review is an introduction to medical, non-cosmetic treatments with botulinum neurotoxin (BoNT) in the orofacial region. It focuses on the current most common, best-documented and safest indications of interest for dentists in terms of dystonia and sialorrhea. These conditions are recommended to start with and suitable to gain better skill and experience with BoNT. The introduction also stresses the importance of correct diagnostics based on interdisciplinary cooperation, precise targeting of the injections, measurements of treatment effect, and control of the oral health with regard to side effects.

Keywords: botulinum toxin; movement disorders; oromandibular dystonia; sialorrhea

Key Contribution: Injections with botulinum toxin guided by electromyography and ultrasonography is a safe, effective, and reversible treatment for orofacial muscle disorders and drooling problems. An interdisciplinary approach and regular control of the oral health are advised.

Citation: Bakke, M. Botulinum Toxin, a Drug with Potential Interest for Dentists—An Introduction. *Toxins* **2022**, *14*, 667. https://doi.org/10.3390/toxins14100667

Received: 8 August 2022
Accepted: 22 September 2022
Published: 25 September 2022

1. Effects of Botulinum Toxin

Botulinum toxin (BoNT) is an extremely toxic substance. The neurotoxin is produced by the bacterium *Clostridium botulinum* under low-oxygen conditions. BoNT is often foodborne, and in the wild, it typically grows in contaminated and improperly stored or poorly prepared foods. In the middle of the last century, it was discovered that even a small dose of BoNT injected intramuscularly could paralyze muscle function locally for several months. Thereafter, the use of BoNT was started for medical purposes, initially to alleviate strabismus and blepharospasms. The use of BoNT has increased significantly since then, not least due to the increasing cosmetic use for wrinkles. In addition to treatment of skeletal muscles, BoNT is used for autonomic disorders [1,2]. Pain treatment has also been initiated, investigated, and performed, especially in relation to neuropathic pain, headaches and migraines [3–5]. Contraindications to BoNT use include a known allergy to BoNT, active inflammation or infection at the proposed injection site, pregnancy, breast-feeding, or chronic degenerative neuromuscular disorders [6].

The background for the therapeutic effects of peripherally administered BoNT on muscle activity and secretion is a prolonged inhibition of the release of the neurotransmitter acetylcholine, an effect that reduces the signal from the nervous system to skeletal muscles and glands. The activity of intrafusal muscle fibers is also inhibited, leading to reduced afferent input from muscle spindles to the central nervous system and thereby contributing to the therapeutic effect [3]. The link between BoNT and pain relief was initially thought to correlate only with its effect on reduced muscle activity in cases with over contraction, cramps or contractures. However, the analgesia provided by BoNT injections occurs before the inhibition of muscle activity, lasts longer than muscle weakness, and has an effect on the nociceptor system [7].

Besides acetylcholine, other chemical messengers may be affected in the injected area, such as glutamate, norepinephrine, serotonin, substance P, calcitonin gene-related peptide and adenosine triphosphate, which may contribute to an antinociceptive effect [3–5]. Retrograde axonal transport may also be involved in the therapeutic effects [8]. It has also been suggested that the BoNT action on pain is dominantly a central effect [9]. However, evidence of an effect by BoNT is still lacking for most pain conditions. Thus in randomized and blinded studies on persistent myofascial temporomandibular disorders; the effect varies from non-existing, uncertain and similar to the effect of conservative treatment with an oral appliance [10–12].

Dentists and dental surgeons have more knowledge than most other health professionals do on anatomy, function, diagnosis and treatment in the orofacial area. Therefore, it seems justified that they use treatment with medical BoNT in this region. However, further skill enhancement to apply BoNT is needed, as well as an interdisciplinary collaboration. Plenty of reports on the use of BoNT in the orofacial area have been published, but at present, quality literature is scarce [13]. However, there are common, safe and generally accepted indications for medical, non-cosmetic treatment with BoNT as shown in Table 1 [2]. In the future, BoNT may also have a role as a supplementary treatment option for conditions in general dentistry where conventional therapy is not always effective, for example, trismus, hypermobility, bruxism and painful masticatory hypertrophy [14–18]. Especially treatment of excessive bruxism may be relevant [19].

Table 1. Common indications for medical BoNT in the orofacial area [2].

Area	Diagnosis	Description
Face	Hemifacial spasm	Irregular, involuntary muscle contractions on one side of the face
	Frey's syndrome (gustatory sweating)	Sweating on the cheek area resulting from damage to or near the parotid gland
Mouth and jaws	Oromandibular dystonia	Involuntary tension or spasm with abnormal movements of the jaw and mouth
	Hypersalivation/sialorrhea	Drooling caused by increased saliva secretion and/or reduced swallowing function

In several countries, treatment with BoNT is limited to a few medical specialties or generally not allowed for dentists, but the interest is still growing. The present overview is intended for dentists as an inspiration to start using these treatments, and it focuses on the effect on orofacial muscle and salivary gland function, which may be the safest to start with.

2. Oromandibular Dystonia (OMD) and Other Movement Disorders in the Oromandibular Area

OMD is a focal movement disorder in the jaw, tongue and mouth, e.g., in the form of involuntary jaw opening and closing, chewing movements and involuntary mouth and tongue movements. It can also present itself as repeated small, but tiring contractions of the jaw muscles during "resting" posture (Figure 1). Accordingly, OMD may inhibit or repress facial expression as well as chewing, swallowing and speech function. When the OMD occurs together with blepharospasm (abnormal contraction of the eyelid muscles), the term Meige's syndrome is often used. The dystonia may be idiopathic, i.e., without any identifiable cause, caused by damage or degeneration of the brain or exposure to particular drugs (tardive).

OMD reduces the quality of life and may cause weight loss, social isolation and depression in patients [14]. Surprisingly, the dystonic muscle activity and the often very strong contractions rarely cause muscle pain, although there may be a feeling of general fatigue. However, when jaw openers are involved, overload and habitual dislocations of the temporomandibular joints may occur, just as the OMD in the jaw closer muscles may traumatize the lips, cheek, tongue and alveolar processes. In addition, the repeated involuntary movements of the mouth and jaws will typically result in severe attrition and damage to the dentition, denture adaptation problems and alveolar atrophy [20]. Therefore, some patients may experience some improvement with the use of oral appliances [21].

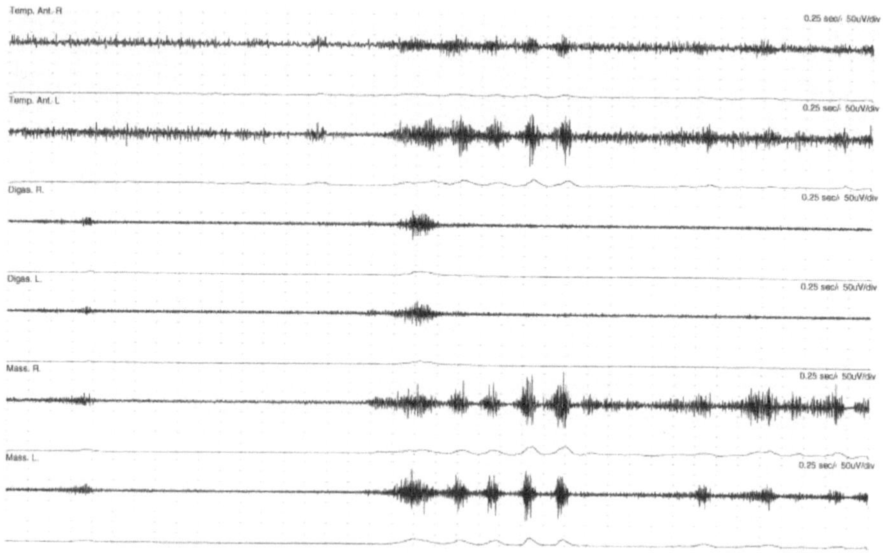

Figure 1. Repeated small but tiring dystonic activity in the jaw muscles during "resting" posture recorded with electromyography and surface electrodes in a female patient with oromandibular dystonia. Marked, synchronous bursts of activity in the anterior temporal (Temp. Ant. R. and L.) and masseter muscles (Mass. R. and L.) with a duration of 0.3–0.5 s, continuous elevated activity in the temporal muscles (Temp. Ant. R. and L.), and little dystonic activity in digastric muscles (Digas. R. and L.).

It may be difficult to recognize OMD, and often patients become misdiagnosed and mistreated, partly due to an overlap between the working areas for dentists and medical specialists and insufficient cooperation [22]. Thus, OMD may also be confused with bruxism. Table 2 illustrates the similarities and differences, and differential diagnoses require neurological, odontological, and anatomical knowledge [22]. There are also other neurological disorders manifesting itself in the orofacial area besides OMD. They are tremor, spasms, cramps or contractures that may arise from disturbances within the nervous systems such as Parkinson's disease (PD) and cerebral palsy (CP), and palliative interventions are indicated to prevent bite wounds in tongue, lips and cheeks in retarded, handicapped or hypermobile persons.

There is no definitive cure for OMD. Currently, BoNT injections are regarded as the treatment of choice for OMD, and there is solid evidence that it is a safe and effective treatment, e.g., [23]. Thus, surveys and meta-analyses of clinical findings have shown that BoNT injections are efficacious in reducing dystonic movements of patients with OMD when properly administered by experienced clinicians [24,25]. The treatment effect with BoNT is temporary. However, with the correct doses and proper identification and treatment of the dystonic muscles, the latency for the full effect after injection of BoNT is about a week, and the effect is optimal within the first 1.5–2 months [2]. Since neuromuscular transmission regenerates slowly, muscle function is restored and the effect ceases after 3–6 months. Therefore, BoNT treatments are typically repeated three to four times per year. Most patients feel significant improvement from the treatment, although they still feel some functional limitations, typically regarding jaw mobility and communication [19]. In the oromandibular region with small muscle groups, vital functions, and delicate anatomical structures, precise injection of the BoNT is crucial [2]. Diffusion at the injection site and spread to unintended areas may lead to significant although short-lasting discomfort. In general, jaw-closing dystonia responds the most robustly while jaw-opening dystonia is more complex to inject, but clinical experience is consistent with benefit [26].

Table 2. Comparison between oromandibular dystonia (OMD) and bruxism [21].

	OMD (ICD-11: 8A02—Dystonic Disorders)	Bruxism (ICD-11: 13DA0E.7—Dentofacial Anomalies)
Main responsible discipline	Neurology	Dentistry
Clinical characteristics	Awake state	Mainly during sleep
Pain	No or only modest tenderness, but fatigue during the day and in the evening	Pain or tenderness of the masticatory muscles and tension headaches, often worst in the morning and on awakening
Dental attrition and trauma	Marked or pathological tooth wear Tooth infractions and fractures Wear or damage to dental restorations	
Provoking factors	Idiopathic or caused by brain damage or drug treatment	Uncertain or physiological and psychosocial factors
Aggravating factors	Psychological stress	
Primary treatment	BoNT and drug treatment	Flat plane stabilizing bite splint
Additional treatment	Flat plane stabilizing bite splint	BoNT

3. Injections of BoNT in the Oromandibular Muscles

Conventional BoNT formulations used in the orofacial area are primarily Botox (onabotulinumtoxinA) and Xenon (incobotulinumtoxinA) and eventually also Dysport (abobotulinumtoxinA) and Myobloc/Neurobloc (botulinumtoxinB). Unlike for other drugs, there is no direct correlation between the dosage units for the various compositions of BoNT, and the formulations are not identical or equivalent for all types [27]. The suggestion of recommended doses for the muscles is shown in Table 3 [2]. However, it is advisable to start with a low dose when treating a muscle in a patient for the first time. In addition, when treating the digastric muscle (anterior belly), the patient should be informed that BoNT injections may cause temporary swallowing difficulties. The treatment is usually repeated 3–4 times per year. Thorough controls are needed so doses and targets can be adjusted if necessary. Controls should also include subjective evaluation on visual analog scales and questionnaires on chewing efficiency and other oral functions to assess the severity of the condition [19]. Note also that repeated BoNT treatment for years may cause bite force as well as muscle atrophy and possibly bone loss [28,29]. See the short-term effect of standard treatment on muscle activity, bite force in a patient with OMD, and marked attrition (Figure 2).

Table 3. Oromandibular muscles, their maximal activation, and recommended doses of BoNT type A (Botox and Xeomin). Units (IU) are shown for one muscle in one side and for the orbicularis oris muscle for each side of the upper and lower part of the lip. Note that the total dose in one session should not exceed 400 IU [2].

Oromandibular Muscles	Maximal Voluntary Contraction	Units of Botox or Xeomin per Muscle and Side
Temporalis Masseter Medial pterygoid	Jaw closing—strong biting	10–45 IU
Digastricus venter anterior	Jaw opening—full mouth opening	5–10 IU
Lateral pterygoid	Jaw opening—side movement and protrusion	10–45 IU
Orbicularis oris	Lip pursing	5–10 IU

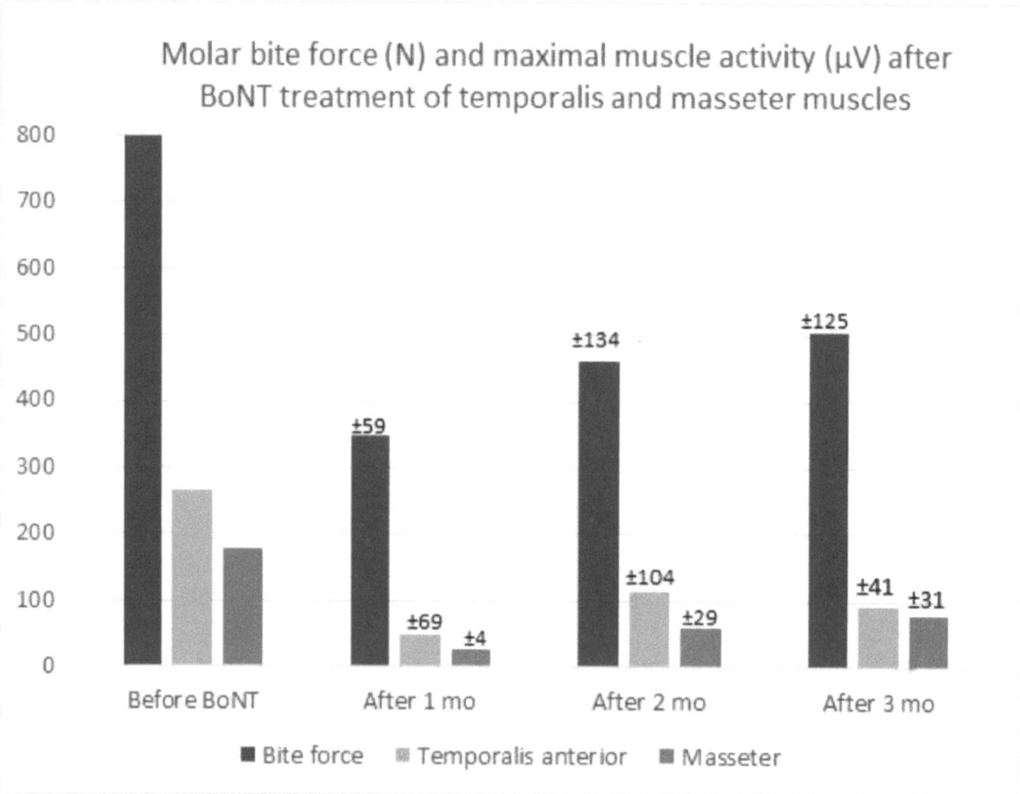

Figure 2. The effect of BoNT-A treatment in a male with jaw-closing dystonia. Bilateral treatment in the anterior temporal and masseter muscles (20–40 IU per muscle as single injections with EMG guidance) on maximal bite force (measured with a unilateral force transducer in the molar region) and the average level of maximal voluntary contraction during biting in the intercuspal position (measured with surface electrodes over the muscles). Values initially before start of first treatment (Before BoNT) and average results (Mean ± SD after 1, 2, and 3 months) from a total of 15 recording sessions (3–4 times per year through 15 years). Note, the marked reduction in values after start of treatment, and also the increase again from 1 month to 2 and 3 months after (muscle function is expected to be restored and the effect ceased after 3–6 months).

Given the potential adverse event of dysphagia and other side effects, one should be cautious while delivering injections. Therefore, many studies employ and recommend electromyography (EMG) or eventually ultrasonographic guidance for muscle targeting. The importance of correct identification and targeting of the affected muscles is the same whether the condition is due to OMD, or contractures, tremor, spasms or cramps. If one is unfamiliar with the possible injection site in these muscles, the procedure becomes easier after checking the locations and the anatomic details of the targeted muscles, and if possible to palpate them during maximal voluntary contraction (see Table 3). Standard disinfection procedures are applied for injection through the skin. The BoNT is best and most safely injected using a cannulated electrode for EMG guidance [2] and reconfirmation of dystonic activity [30]. It is stated that from the point of injection the BoNT diffuses 1 to 1.5 cm [31]. The reported number of injection sites may vary from one to five sites per muscle, e.g., [30,31]. For small muscles, a bolus injection will do nicely [31]. Few injection sites also means less superficial reddening and pain of the skin in relation to the treatment.

Before administration, the correct placement of the cannulated needle electrode can be confirmed by the presence of an interference pattern during maximal effort of the muscle and the dystonia by involuntary activity during rest. Without such precautions, the BoNT may be misplaced and treatment intended for masseter may give dryness of the mouth because of the close relation to the parotid gland.

The site for the percutaneous injections are for the masseter the lower half of the superficial part, for the temporalis muscle the anterior voluminous part, for the medial (internal) pterygoid muscle on the medial side of the ramus just above its fusion with the sling with the masseter, and for the digastric muscle the anterior belly. With respect to the orbicularis oris muscles, the injection is in the protruding parts but just above (upper lip) and below (lower lip) the carmine red margin of the lip. The lateral (external) pterygoid is best approached intraorally to have direct access for palpation and injection. The direction of the needle insertion is posteriorly and slightly laterally in parallel with the buccal surfaces of the maxillary molars.

4. Saliva Secretion and Sialorrhea

Under normal physiological conditions, saliva secretion amounts to about 1–1.5 L per day. There is higher secretion rates during chewing and with taste stimulation than at rest [32] and people usually swallow the saliva unconsciously. The unstimulated, resting secretion rate of whole saliva is 0.2–0.5 mL per min during wakefulness and practically negligible during sleep. The most important salivary glands are the parotid and the submandibular glands, which produce most of the saliva, e.g., [33]. These major glands have different functional patterns. The saliva during stimulation is predominantly secreted by the parotid glands situated in close relation and lateral to the masseter muscles. The unstimulated saliva during rest is mainly produced by the submandibular glands at the inner surface of the mandibular corpus.

Sialorrhea or drooling is characterized by the inability to control oral secretions, resulting in excessive saliva in the oropharynx and unintentional loss of saliva from the mouth. It takes place in the daytime outside meals, and is unusual in healthy subjects after the age of 5 years. Sialorrhea is frequent in neurological patients and is considered a great clinical and social handicap. It can be classified either as mainly anterior, i.e., over the lip margin when insufficient closure causes overflow of saliva from the mouth, or posterior, i.e., with aspiration, coughing and risk of lung inflammation [34]. Severe drooling may also cause skin irritation around the mouth. A great number of napkins, bibs, scarfs, handkerchiefs, and paper towels may be needed to wipe away saliva from the mouth and chin and to keep the clothes dry. This effect of drooling is often associated with reduced quality of life with discomfort, limitations in activities and social embarrassment.

Rather than regular hypersalivation (so-called primary sialorrhea), the accumulation of saliva in the mouth is most often due to decreased swallowing function (secondary sialorrhea), and may even be present with low salivary flow rates. Primary sialorrhea is often related to gastroesophageal reflux, pregnancy, or develops as a side effect of pharmacological treatment [2]. In contrast, neurodegenerative diseases, such as amyotrophic lateral sclerosis and PD, often cause secondary sialorrhea as they affect the swallowing centers in the medulla and pontine area, the motor neurons, or the cortical and subcortical centers initiating or regulating swallowing.

5. Treatment of Sialorrhea with BoNT

Sialorrhea has previously been treated with methods that are either quite ineffective, such as exercise or very invasive, such as surgery or radiation. In contrast, BoNT is now a very promising and reversible treatment, but must be repeated at regular intervals. By injections with Botox in each parotid (25–40 IU) and each submandibular (15–30 IU) both drooling and flow can be reduced 2 weeks after treatment with maximal reductions of 30–40% [33].

Through intraglandular injection of BoNT into the larger salivary glands, a blockade occurs in the neurogenic (parasympathetic) control of salivary secretion approximately at one week post-injection, and persists 3–6 months, i.e., similar to the duration of the effect of BoNT treatment in the muscles [3]. However, it is essential that the relevant glands are targeted accurately. Although this may be achieved by using anatomical landmarks, the use of ultrasonographic guidance seems preferable to increase the treatment safety. In the hands of a trained injector, this technique is a quick and non-invasive imaging technique to identify the correct site [35]. Before the treatment start, it is important to record the frequency and extent of the drooling as well as the impact of the drooling problems. The pre- and posttreatment assessment of drooling should include measurement of the unstimulated salivary secretion rate together with a classification of drooling, e.g., by Thomas-Stonell and Greenberg [36], for severity combined and frequency. The number of used bibs, paper towels and handkerchiefs per day or week is good supplementary documentation of the treatment effect.

A recent large prospective, randomized, double-blind, and placebo-controlled multicenter study has clearly demonstrated that 100 IU Xeomin, i.e., each parotid gland 30 IU and each submandibular gland 20 IU, is an effective and well-tolerated treatment of chronic sialorrhea in adult patients [37]. There was a significant reduction in the unstimulated salivary flow rate at week 4, which was also significant different compared with placebo. In addition, the side effects were few, i.e., 3–5% dry mouth and 0–3% dysphagia (Table 4).

Table 4. Reports on BoNT treatments of chronic sialorrhea.

Authors	Study Type	Patients	Glands (BoNT)	Guidance
Jost, Friedman, Michel et al., 2019 [35]	Randomized, placebo-controlled, double-blind study	Adults with PD, parkinsonism, stroke, or traumatic brain injury	Parotid 30 IU bilaterally + submandibular 20 IU bilaterally (all Xeomin)	All with ultrasonic guidance
Ruiz-Roca, Pons-Fuster and Lopez-Jorne, 2019 [38]	Systematic review of 21 studies	Mainly elderly with PD	Most cases both parotid + submandibular (mainly BoNT-A, no consensus on doses or type of BoNT)	43% with ultrasonic guidance, else anatomical landmarks or palpation
Hung, Liao, Lin et al., 2021 [39]	Systematic review and meta-analysis of 21 studies	Children with CP	62% both parotid + submandibular bilaterally (90% Botox, no consensus on doses, but should not exceed 4 IU/kg)	81% with ultrasonic guidance

In a systematic review on adults with PD all 21 studies showed a reduction in sialorrhea, but no consensus regarding the site of injection of the toxin (single or multiple points) or toxin dose [39]. A similar review based on 21 studies in children with CP found likewise, that BoNT-A injections (mainly with Botox and ultrasound) are a safe, reversible, effective treatment for drooling in children, even if doses and target glands varied, except that the total dosage should not exceed 4 IU/kg [40].

In the short term, the side effects from intraglandular BoNT injections were few in the reports. However, changes in the salivary viscosity have been reported as the total protein and amylase concentration generally increases with decreasing flow [33,41]. Thus, the saliva changes from being mainly watery and clear to sticky and frothy. This may be important over time, as saliva plays a significant role in keeping the relationship between the host and oral microbiota in a symbiotic state 8n the mouth and as the natural balance of the oral microbiome is often disturbed in conditions with salivary gland dysfunction, leading to gingivitis, caries, and fungal infection [41]. Therefore, similar changes could be expected with BoNT-treatment for many years, but there is currently insufficient evidence [42]. Only small changes in the saliva have been found in patients successfully treated with BoNT such as increased level of *Lactobacilli* and amylase [32,43]. However, because of the possible risk in the long term patients with intraglandular BoNT injections should have regularly dental control to prevent and treat possible oral side effects.

6. Conclusions

With their theoretical and practical background, dentists are able to carry out injections with BoNT after supplementary training and according to the various national guidelines and approvals. Several medical conditions in the oromandibular region may benefit from such treatment. Presently, in the area of responsibility for dentists, the conditions are primarily muscle disorders and drooling problems, in which the use of BoNT is safe, effective, and reversible. These health disorders and problems are generally not associated with pain, but with disabilities of oral function, embarrassment, and severely reduced quality of life.

Interdisciplinary collaboration between dentists and neurologist and/or otologists is important for precise diagnostics and treatment. As supplement to the clinical investigation of the muscle disorders EMG recordings are relevant to assess more accurately, which muscles are involved and which abnormalities are present. For sialorrhea, measurement of the unstimulated secretion is relevant for the assessment of type and for later control. To achieve the best results and minimize or prevent side effects, use standard doses, guidance of the BoNT injections with EMG or ultrasonography, and regular and standardized treatments and controls.

Funding: This research received no external funding.

Institutional Review Board Statement: Not applicable.

Informed Consent Statement: Not applicable.

Data Availability Statement: Not applicable.

Conflicts of Interest: The author declares no conflict of interest.

Abbreviations

BoNT	botulinum toxin
Botox	onabotulinumtoxinA
CP	cerebral palsy
EMG	electromyography
Myobloc/neurobloc	botulinumtoxinB
OMD	oromandibular disorders
Xenon	incobotulinumtoxinA
PD	Parkinson's disease

References

1. Bakke, M.; Møller, E.; Dalager, T. Botulinum toxin—Et lægemiddel af potentiel interesse for tandlæger. *Tandlaegebladet* **2013**, *117*, 894–899.
2. Bakke, M.; Dalager, T.; Møller, E. What clinical strategies are applied for botulinum toxin injection in the oromandibular region? In *Botulinum Toxin Therapy Manual for Dystonia and Spasticity*; Rosales, R., Dressler, D., Eds.; InTech: Rijeka, Croatia, 2016; pp. 79–95.
3. Pirazzini, M.; Rossetto, O.; Eleopra, R.; Montecucco, C. Botulinum neurotoxins: Biology, pharmacology, and toxicology. *Pharmacol. Rev.* **2017**, *69*, 200–235. [CrossRef]
4. Park, J.; Park, J.P. Botulinum toxin for the treatment of neuropathic pain. *Toxins* **2017**, *9*, 260. [CrossRef]
5. Sandrini, G.; De Icco, R.; Tassorelli, C.; Smania, N.; Tamburin, S. Botulinum neurotoxin type A for the treatment of pain: Not just in migraine and trigeminal neuralgia. *J. Headache Pain* **2017**, *18*, 38. [CrossRef] [PubMed]
6. Mor, N.; Tang, C.; Blitzer, A. Temporomandibular myofacial pain treated with botulinum toxin injection. *Toxins* **2015**, *7*, 2791–2800. [CrossRef] [PubMed]
7. Wheeler, A.; Smith, H.S. Botulinum toxins: Mechanisms of action, antinociception and clinical applications. *Toxicology* **2013**, *306*, 124–146. [CrossRef]
8. Waskitho, A.; Yamamoto, Y.; Raman, S.; Kano, F.; Yan, H.; Raju, R.; Afroz, S.; Morita, T.; Ikutame, D.; Okura, K.; et al. Peripherally administered botulinum toxin type A localizes bilaterally in trigeminal ganglia of animal model. *Toxins* **2021**, *13*, 704. [CrossRef]

9. Matak, I.; Lackovic, Z. Botulinum toxin A, brain and pain. *Prog. Neurobiol.* **2014**, *119–120*, 39–59. [CrossRef]
10. Ernberg, M.; Hedenberg-Magnusson, B.; List, T.; Svensson, P. Efficacy of botulinum toxin type A for treatment of persistent myofascial TMD pain: A randomized, controlled, double-blind multicenter study. *Pain* **2011**, *152*, 1988–1996. [CrossRef]
11. Machado, D.; Martimbianco, A.L.C.; Bussadori, S.K.; Pacheco, R.L.; Riera, R.; Santos, E.M. Botulinum Toxin Type A for painful temporomandibular disorders: Systematic review and meta-analysis. *J. Pain* **2020**, *21*, 281–293. [CrossRef]
12. De la Torre Canales, G.; Alvarez-Pinzon, N.; Muñoz-Lora, V.R.M.; Peroni, L.V.; Gomes, A.F.; Sánchez-Ayala, A.; Haiter-Neto, F.; Manfredini, D.; Rizzatti-Barbosa, C.M. Efficacy and safety of botulinum toxin type A on persistent myofascial pain: A randomized clinical trial. *Toxins* **2020**, *12*, 395. [CrossRef] [PubMed]
13. Srivastava, S.; Kharbanda, S.; Pal, U.S.; Shah, V. Application of botulinum toxin in dentistry: A comprehensive review. *Natl. J. Maxillofac. Surg.* **2015**, *6*, 152–159.
14. Bakke, M.; Baram, S.; Dalager, T.; Biernat, H.B.; Møller, E. Oromandibular dystonia, mental distress and oro-facial dysfunction—A follow-up 8–10 years after start of treatment with botulinum toxin. *J. Oral Rehabil.* **2019**, *46*, 441–449. [CrossRef] [PubMed]
15. Bakke, M.; Møller, E.; Werdelin, L.M.; Dalager, T.; Kitai, N.; Kreiborg, S. Treatment of severe temporomandibular joint clicking with botulinum toxin in the lateral pterygoid muscle in two cases of anterior disc displacement. *Oral Surg. Oral Med. Oral Pathol. Oral Radiol. Endod.* **2005**, *100*, 693–700. [CrossRef]
16. Møller, E.; Bakke, M.; Dalager, T.; Werdelin, L.M. Oromandibular dystonia involving the lateral pterygoid muscles: Four cases with different complexity. *Mov. Disord.* **2007**, *22*, 785–790. [CrossRef]
17. Yoshida, K. Botulinum neurotoxin injection for the treatment of recurrent temporomandibular joint dislocation with and without neurogenic muscular hyperactivity. *Toxins* **2018**, *10*, 174. [CrossRef] [PubMed]
18. Yoshida, K. Effects of botulinum toxin type A on pain among trigeminal neuralgia, myofascial temporomandibular disorders, and oromandibular dystonia. *Toxins* **2021**, *13*, 605. [CrossRef]
19. Long, H.; Liao, Z.; Wang, Y.; Liao, L.; Lai, W. Efficacy of botulinum toxins on bruxism: An evidence-based review. Efficacy of botulinum toxins on bruxism: An evidence-based review. *Int. Dent. J.* **2012**, *62*, 1–5. [CrossRef]
20. Bakke, M.; Larsen, B.M.; Dalager, T.; Møller, E. Oromandibular dystonia—Functional and clinical characteristics: A report on 21 cases. *Oral Surg. Oral Med. Oral Pathol. Oral Radiol.* **2013**, *115*, e21–e26. [CrossRef]
21. De Meyer, M.; Vereecke, L.; Bottenberg, P.; Jacquet, W.; Sims, A.B.; Santens, P. Oral appliances in the treatment of oromandibular dystonia: A systematic review. *Acta Neurol. Belg.* **2020**, *120*, 831–836. [CrossRef]
22. Kjelde, A.B.T.; Rasmussen, H.S.; Bakke, M. Oromandibulær dystoni. *Tandlaegebladet* **2021**, *125*, 658–663.
23. Tan, E.K.; Jankovic, J. Botulinum toxin A in patients with oromandibular dystonia: Long-term follow-up. *Neurology* **1999**, *53*, 2102–2107. [CrossRef]
24. Yoshida, K. Botulinum toxin therapy for oromandibular dystonia and other movement disorders in the stomatognathic system. *Toxins* **2022**, *14*, 282. [CrossRef]
25. Dadgardoust, P.D.; Rosales, R.L.; Asuncion, R.M.; Dressler, D. Botulinum neurotoxin a therapy efficacy and safety for oromandibular dystonia: A meta-analysis. *J. Neural Transm.* **2019**, *126*, 141–148. [CrossRef]
26. Comella, C.L. Systematic review of botulinum toxin treatment for oromandibular dystonia. *Toxicon* **2018**, *147*, 96–99. [CrossRef] [PubMed]
27. Choudhury, S.; Baker, M.R.; Chatterjee, S.; Hrishikesh, K. Botulinum toxin: An update on pharmacology and newer products in development. *Toxins* **2021**, *13*, 58. [CrossRef]
28. Balanta-Melo, J.; Toto-Ibacache, V.; Kupczik, K.; Buvinic, S. Mandibular bone loss after masticatory muscles intervention with botulinum toxin: An approach from basic research to clinical findings. *Toxins* **2019**, *11*, 84. [CrossRef] [PubMed]
29. Kahn, A.; Kün-Darbois, J.D.; Bertin, H.; Corre, P.; Chappard, D. Mandibular bone effects of botulinum toxin injections in masticatory muscles in adult. *Oral Surg. Oral Med. Oral Pathol. Oral Radiol.* **2020**, *129*, 100–108. [CrossRef]
30. Møller, E.; Werdelin, L.M.; Bakke, M.; Dalager, T.; Prytz, S.; Regeur, L. Treatment of perioral dystonia with botulinum toxin in 4 cases of Meige's syndrome. *Oral Surg. Oral Med. Oral Pathol. Oral Radiol. Endod.* **2003**, *96*, 544–549. [CrossRef]
31. Sinclair, C.F.; Gurey, L.E.; Blitzer, A. Oromandibular dystonia: Long-term management with botulinum toxin. *Laryngoscope* **2013**, *123*, 3078–3083. [CrossRef] [PubMed]
32. Jost, W.H.; Baümer, T.; Laskaw, R.; Slawek, J.; Spittau, B.; Steffen, A.; Winterholler, M.; Bavikatte, G. Therapy of sialorrhea with botulinum neurotoxin. *Neurol. Ther.* **2019**, *8*, 273–288. [CrossRef] [PubMed]
33. Møller, E.; Karlsborg, M.; Bardow, A.; Lykkeaa, J.; Nissen, F.H.; Bakke, M. Treatment of severe drooling with botulinum toxin in amyotrophic lateral sclerosis and Parkinson's disease: Efficacy and possible mechanisms. *Acta Odont. Scand.* **2011**, *69*, 151–157. [CrossRef] [PubMed]
34. Bakke, M.; Bardow, A.; Møller, E. Severe drooling and treatment with botulinum toxin. *Perspect. Swallowing Swallowing Disord. (Dysphagia)* **2012**, *21*, 15–21. [CrossRef]
35. Jost, W.H. The option of sonographic guidance in botulinum toxin injection for drooling in Parkinson's disease. *J. Neural. Transm.* **2016**, *123*, 51–55. [CrossRef]
36. Thomas-Stonell, N.; Greenberg, S.J. Three treatment approaches and clinical factors in the reduction of drooling. *Dysphagia* **1988**, *3*, 73–78. [CrossRef] [PubMed]
37. Jost, W.H.; Friedman, A.; Michel, O.; Oehlwein, C.; Slawek, J.; Bogucki, A.; Ochudlo, S.; Banach, M.; Pagan, F.; Flatau-Baqué, B.; et al. Placebo-controlled, randomized, double-blind study of incobotulinumtoxin A for sialorrhea. *Neurology* **2019**, *92*, e1982–e1991. [CrossRef]

38. Ruiz-Roca, J.A.; Pons-Fuster, E.; Lopez-Jorne, P. Effectiveness of the botulinum toxin for treating sialorrhea in patients with Parkinson's disease: A systematic review. *J. Clin. Med.* **2019**, *8*, 317. [CrossRef]
39. Hung, S.A.; Liao, C.L.; Lin, W.P.; Hsu, J.C.; Guo, Y.H.; Lin, Y.C. Botulinum toxin injections for treatment of drooling in children with cerebral palsy: A systematic review and meta-analysis. *Children* **2021**, *8*, 1089. [CrossRef]
40. Tiigimäe-Saar, J.; Taba, P.; Tamme, T. Does the botulinum neuro-toxin type A treatment for sialorrhea change oral health? *Clin. Oral Investig.* **2017**, *21*, 795–800. [CrossRef]
41. Lynge Pedersen, A.M.; Belstrøm, D. The role of natural salivary defences in maintaining a healthy oral microbiota. *J. Dent.* **2019**, *80* (Suppl. S1), S3–S12. [CrossRef]
42. Correa, L.B.; Basso, M.B.; Tiigimäe-Saar Sousa-Pinto, B.; Leal, S.C. Oral health effects of botulinum toxin treatment for drooling: A systematic review. *Med. Oral Patol. Oral Cir. Bucal.* **2021**, *26*, e172–e180. [CrossRef] [PubMed]
43. Tiigimäe-Saar, J.; Tamme, T.; Rosenthal, M.; Kadastik-Eerme, L.; Taba, P. Saliva changes in Parkinson's disease patients after injection of botulinum neurotoxin type A. *Neurol. Sci.* **2018**, *39*, 871–877. [CrossRef] [PubMed]

toxins

MDPI

Review

Botulinum Toxin—A Current Place in the Treatment of Chronic Migraine and Other Primary Headaches

Katarzyna Kępczyńska * and Izabela Domitrz

Department of Neurology, Medical University of Warsaw, 80 Cegłowska St., 01-809 Warsaw, Poland
* Correspondence: kkepczynska@wum.edu.pl

Abstract: Headaches are a very common condition that most people will experience many times during their lives. This article presents the primary headaches, which are a large group of diseases where the headache is not a symptom of another known disease. Tension-type headache affects approximately 80% of the general population, and the prevalence of migraine is estimated at 10–12%. Clinical data and experience to date have demonstrated that botulinum toxin may be an effective prophylactic treatment for chronic headache types. It has been used in neurology for the treatment of dystonia and blepharospasm. Now it has been approved to treat chronic migraine and has been shown to confer significant benefit in refractory cases. Based on clinical experience botulinum toxin has also been tried in other headache disorders. While it is intuitively attractive to think that due to its effect on pain by sensory modulation, there may also be efficacy in its use in chronic tension-type headache and cluster headache, so far, there is little evidence to support this. Botulinum toxin is effective in pain control through its interaction with the SNARE complex, which inhibits the release of neurotransmitters, such as glutamate, substance P and calcitonin gene-related peptide. OnabotulinumtoxinA is effective not only in headache frequency and pain intensity but in other parameters, including quality of life.

Keywords: chronic migraine; tension-type headache; cluster headache; onabotulinumtoxinA; headaches; botulinum toxin

Key Contribution: This review highlights the role of botulinum toxin in the threatment of chronic migraine and other primary headaches. Botulinum toxin is clinically used as an attractive alternative for patients who do not respond to other drugs.

Citation: Kępczyńska, K.; Domitrz, I. Botulinum Toxin—A Current Place in the Treatment of Chronic Migraine and Other Primary Headaches. *Toxins* **2022**, *14*, 619. https://doi.org/10.3390/toxins14090619

Received: 17 August 2022
Accepted: 1 September 2022
Published: 5 September 2022

1. Introduction

Headaches are a very common condition that most people will experience many times during their lives. The World Health Organization (WHO) estimated that almost half of all adults will have experienced at least one headache within the last year. There are several kinds of headaches caused by various factors such as our environment, the medication we take and other causes. The International Classification of Headache Disorders 3rd edition (ICHD-3) defines more than 150 different types of headaches, which it divides into two main categories: primary and secondary [1]. The primary headaches, otherwise named idiopathic, are a large group of diseases and syndromes in which the etiology is unclear, and the headache is not a symptom of another known disease. The most common of these are migraines, tension-type headaches and trigeminal autonomic cephalalgias. On the other hand, secondary headaches may be a symptom of a serious underlying medical condition [2].

Migraines are highly prevalent. As a chronic disease, it is the third most common and the seventh most disabling illness globally in people under 50 years old [3]. Only correct diagnosis and effective treatment positively affect a patient's quality of life. Chronic migraine (CM) is defined by the current ICHD- 3 as a headache occurring on ≥15 days per month for 3 months with features of migraine on ≥8 days/month and is a disabling condition that effects 0.5% to 5% of the general population [1]. The progression of episodic migraine to chronic migraine is a complex mechanism that is not fully understood. However, known modifiable risk factors for the progression include the frequency of headache attacks, stressful life events and ineffective acute treatment [4].

There are many treatment options available to help manage the pain. Pharmacologic management for primary headaches includes both: acute and prophylactic treatment strategies. However, we often observe considerable side effects with these therapies, which, unfortunately, limits their usefulness. In patients who take medications too often to treat their headaches, MOH—Medication Overuse Headache—may occur. It is also known as a rebound headache. These can cause migraine episodes to occur more frequently and become more severe. Instead of alleviating symptoms, the medications increase the intensity and frequency of headaches [5]. Migraines, if it is not effectively managed, can lead to significant disability. The primary goals of migraine treatment include relieving the pain, reducing headache frequency and preventing progression to chronic migraine.

Migraines are often refractory to medical therapy and may respond well to onabotulinum toxin (ONABoNTA). ONA-BoNTA is used in neurology for the treatment of dystonia and blepharospasm. Now ONA-BoNTA injections are approved for preventing chronic migraines. The clinical efficacy of botulinum toxin serotype A has been shown in two phase III, placebo-controlled trials (PREEMPT 1 and PREEMPT 2) [6,7]. Based on the phase III program, the number of headache days per month was significantly lower. Significant reductions in the frequency of headache days, headache episodes and triptane use were observed. In summary, the authors noted that OnabotulinumtoxinA positively influenced quality of life and had an acceptable safety profile.

2. Clinical History of Botulinum Toxin

BoNT is a neurotoxin produced by the bacteria Clostridium botulinum. This neurotoxin is responsible for botulism. It inhibits the release of the acetylcholine neurotransmitter from axon endings at the neuromuscular junction. There are eight types of BoNT: from A to H. Types A and B are used in headache treatment. The history of the botulinum toxin is long and interesting. The beginning of the history of botulinum toxin began in 1820 when Justinus Kerner published a description of botulism. In 1897, a group of 34 Belgian musicians consumed smoked ham and developed visual and gastrointestinal symptoms characteristic of botulism. The remaining ham was sent to Professor van Ermengem at the University of Ghent. He found the reason for those symptoms, an agent named Bacillus botulinum, though the name was later changed to Clostridium botulinum [8,9]. The clinical use of BoNT began when Dr. Alan Scott used the toxin botulinum in strabismus. Next, the Food and Drug Administration (FDA) approved conducting human research using the toxin for the treatment of strabismus. In 1989, the FDA approved the use of the toxin for the treatment of blepharospasm and hemifacial spasm. One year later, a facial plastic surgeon Dr. Binder observed that some patients who were administered botulinum toxin for cosmetic purposes reported reduced headache frequency. Prospective open-label observational studies confirmed the acceptable safety and tolerability profile of ONA-BoNTA in chronic migraine prophylaxis [10]. In 2010, ONA-BoNTA was reported as effective for the treatment of chronic migraine in the Phase 3 Research Evaluating Migraine Prophylaxis Therapy (PREEMPT) trials [6,7]. Next, it was approved by the European Medicines Agency (EMA) and by the US Food and Drug Administration (FDA) for the prophylaxis of chronic migraines. Its use was endorsed by the National Institute for Health and Care Excellence (NICE) in 2012.

3. Tension-Type Headache

Nowadays, ONA-BoNTA is only approved to treat CM. Moreover, it has effects on pain by sensory modulation, therefore, it may also be effective for chronic tension-type headache (CTTH). Tension-type headache (TTH) is another condition with a very high socio-economic consequence. It affects approximately 80% of the general population. The pain in TTH is usually bilateral and is not accompanied by other symptoms [1,11]. TTH affects the temporal and occipital region. CTTH is defined as the occurrence of tension-type headaches at a frequency of ≥15 days per month. Tension-type headache treatment should be multilevel. It often consists of taking pain medication, antidepressants, antiepileptics, acupuncture and attending behavioral therapy. The proposed mechanism of the effect of BoNT in chronic tension-type headaches is the reduction in pericranial muscle tension. It should be emphasized that according to ICHD-3 [1], TTH is divided into two types: those with and those without increased pericranial tenderness upon manual palpation. Not every case of TTH is associated with increased muscle tension, and the name may also suggest "mental and emotional tension". Pihut et al. [12] suggested that TTH is, in many cases, related to excessive and long-lasting tension within the muscles of the temporomandibular joint. After the injections of botulinum toxin type A, the character of TTH changed, and its intensity decreased. Moreover, a decrease in the daily number of hours and the monthly number of days was also observed [12]. However, there are also studies that do not support the assertion between the use of BoNT and reduction in TTH pain [13–15]. To sum up, the currently available scientific data on the efficacy of botulinum toxin in tension-type headaches is ambiguous. BoNT as a potent muscle relaxant may be useful in the treatment of TTH, but these assumptions should be confirmed in large groups of TTH patients. In fact, the pathogenesis of TTH as an idiopathic headache is not related to capillary muscle tone, but the pain is receptor-based and central, although it is not fully understood. More positive results will allow for such a course of action to be recommended. It is worth noting that there are sometimes situations where patients who were initially diagnosed with TTH, after careful history taking, will have the diagnosis adjusted to chronic migraine. BoNT in that situation may be beneficial [16].

4. The Use of Botulinum Toxin for the Treatment of Cluster Headache

A cluster headache is a trigeminal autonomic cephalalgia characterized by an extremely painful, strictly unilateral, short-lasting headache attack accompanied by ipsilateral autonomic symptoms. The severity of the disorder has major effects on the patient's quality of life. The most effective drugs to treat an acute cluster headache attack include 100% oxygen inhalation and triptans sc [17,18]. The efficiency of botulinum toxin in cluster headaches was only observed in some studies [19,20]. Botulinum toxin was administered to the spheno-palatine ganglion and the number of cluster headache attacks was significantly reduced [19]. Another pilot study by Crespi et al. suggested that injection with BoNT to the otic ganglion did not reduce the number of attacks per week 2 months after injection. Perhaps this injection location is not an important target in the treatment of chronic cluster headaches [21]. The injection into the spheno-palatine ganglion is a much more complex procedure than the procedure used for chronic migraine. In practice, botulinum toxin is not used in the treatment of cluster headaches. Further studies are warranted to establish the potential of this possible novel treatment for cluster headaches.

5. Botulinum Toxin in the Management of Chronic Migraine

According to the ICHD-3, the diagnosis of chronic migraine was mentioned above. Moreover, the diagnosis of chronic migraine is based on the patient's history (including a headache diary) and neurological examination. To rule out secondary causes for headaches, magnetic resonance of the brain and lumbar puncture may be necessary. The main goal in the treatment of chronic migraine is to reduce the impact of migraines on patients' lives [22]. It is very important to keep migraine attacks as rare, short and as least impairing as possible. There are two pillars for the treatment of chronic migraine: treatment of acute attacks and prophylactic treatment. Due to the risk of MOH, prophylactic treatment is important in this group of patients. The overuse of headache medications can be a problem for patients with chronic headache disorders. One of the substances approved by the United States Food and Drug Administration for the treatment of CM, as mentioned before, is ONA-BoNTA [10,23].

Over the years, several studies failed to indicate the positive effects of BoNT on episodic migraines [16,24]. For chronic migraines, the results were inconsistent. All patients responded to the treatment of botulinum toxin type A, but this response was not superior to the placebo [25,26].

A breakthrough in the use of ONA-BoNTA in the treatment of chronic migraine came in 2010. There were two studies: PREEMPT I and PREEMPT II (Phase III Research Evaluating Migraine Prophylaxis Therapy), in which a total of 1384 patients were enrolled [6,7]. In these two studies (PREEMPT I and II), all patients received a minimum intramuscular dose of 155 units of ONA-BoNTA administered to 31 injection sites across seven head and neck muscles using a fixed side. The minimum dose was 155 units, and the maximum dose was 195 units. The main results from the PREEMPT clinical program have established that ONA-BoNTA is a safe, well-tolerated and effective headache prophylactic treatment for CM [6,7,27]. PREEMPT results support previous studies, which identified chronic migraine patients as most likely to benefit from ONA-BoNTA treatment [25,26,28]. ONA-BoNTA dosing for CM by muscle using the PRREMPT injection program is shown in Table 1. When deciding on the dose and location of additional onabotulinumtoxin type A, the location of the patient's predominant pain and the severity is important.

Table 1. OnabotulinumtoxinA dosing in chronic migraine according to protocol PRREMPT [24].

Area of Injection	Recommended Dose
Frontalis	20 units (4 sites)
Corrugator	10 units (2 sites)
Procerus	5 units (1 site)
Occipitalis	30 units (6 sites) + 10 units in 2 sites (follow the pain areas—optional injections)
Temporalis	40 units (8 sites) + 10 units in 2 sites (follow the pain areas—optional injections)
Trapezius	30 units (6 sites) + 20 units in 4 sites (follow the pain areas—optional injections)
Cervical paraspinal muscle group	20 units (4 sites)
	Summary: 155–195 units

Retreatment with botulinum toxin occurs at 12-week intervals. Meanwhile, patients should keep a headache diary. It is recommended to repeat the injection every 12 months, at least three times. Moreover, the patient should receive additional injections in areas where, in particular, they have pain. This additional treatment strategy is called "Follow the pain", and it was also used by many of the PRREMPT testing sites before FDA approval. Injection points of the botulinum toxin are presented in Figures 1–3, where a patient with chronic migraine who was treated with botulinum toxin with a positive therapeutic effect is shown.

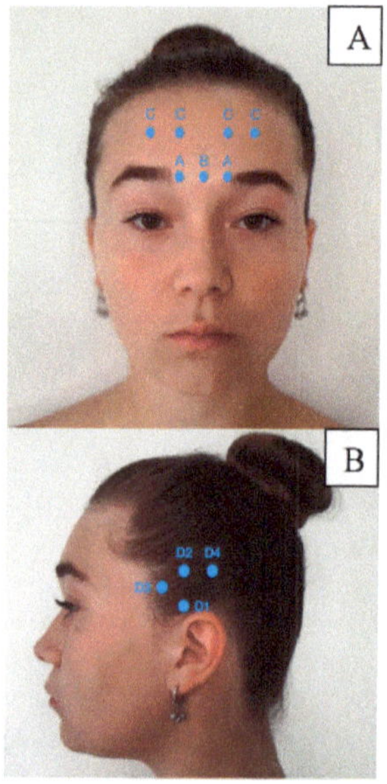

A

A. Corrugator (5 units each side)

B. Procerus (5 units)

C. Frontalis (10 units each side)

B

D1–D4. Temporalis (20 units each side)

Figure 1. Frontalis and temporalis injections of botulinum toxin.

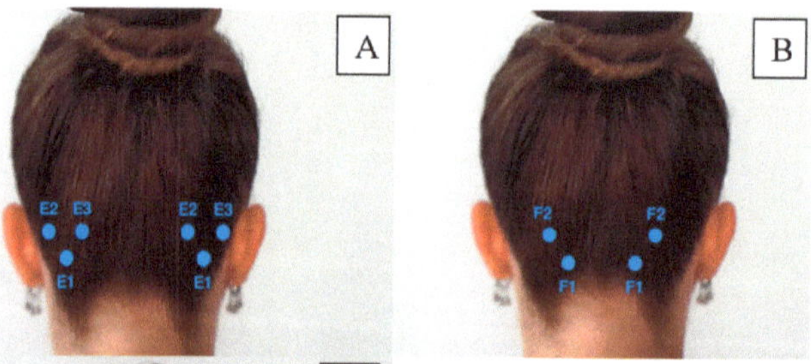

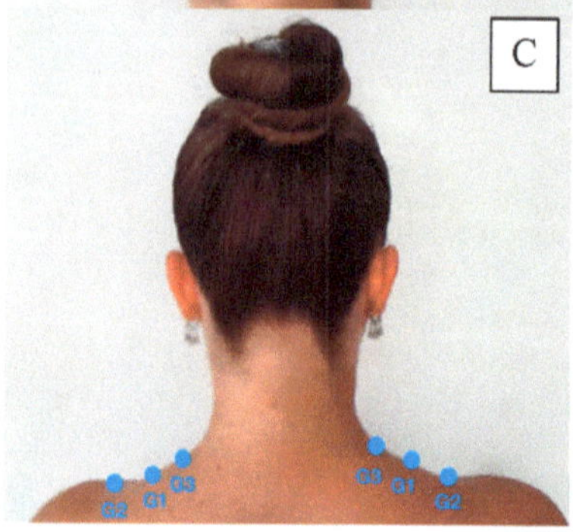

A. E1–E3. Occipitalis (15 units each side)

B. F1–F2. Cervical paraspinal (10 units each side)

C. G1–G3. Trapezius (15 units each side)

Figure 2. Posterior injections of botulinum toxin.

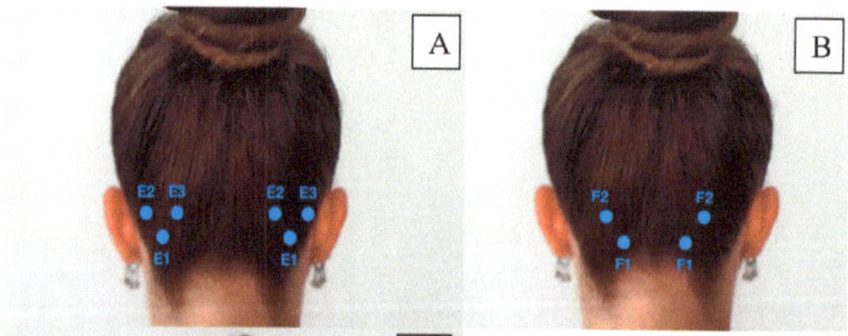

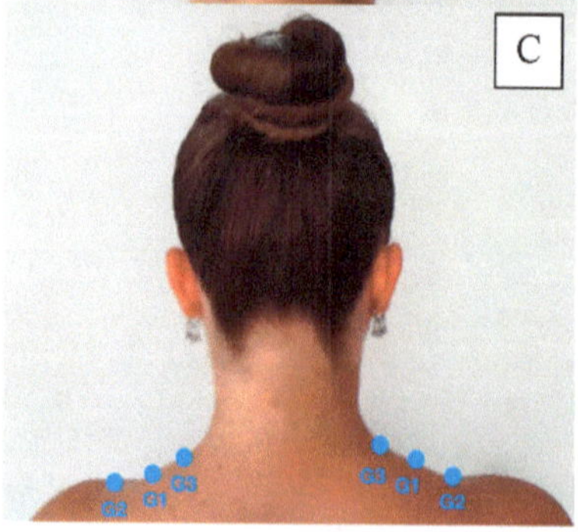

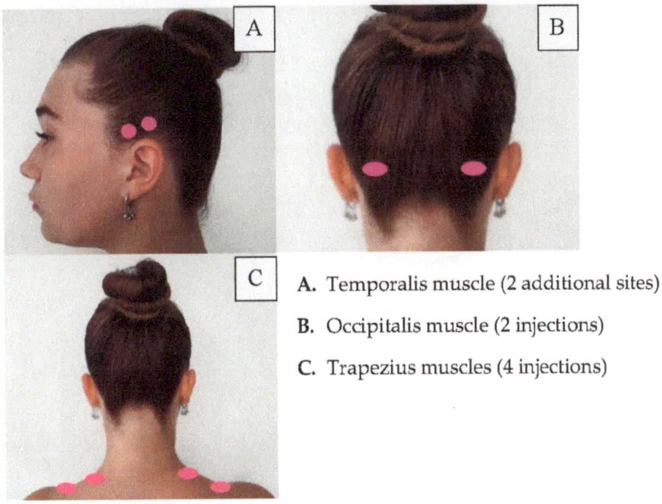

Figure 3. Follow the pain injection sites.

6. Mode of Action of ONA-BoNTA

When onabotulinumtoxin type A is injected into the extracellular space, the heavy chain of the toxin binds to receptors on the C-fiber nerve terminal. Then, ONA-BoNTA is endocytosed and enters the nerve terminal enclosed in a vesicle. Next, botulinum toxin uses its endopeptidase light chain to deactivate the synaptosomal protein known as SNAP-25. This protein is located on the cell membrane, and its deactivation prevents the release of acetylcholine. Moreover, CGRP calcitonin gene-related peptide and other neuropeptides cannot be released [8,23,29,30]. The ability of ONA-BoNTA to block CGRP is likely critical to its therapeutic role in migraines. More recent studies show that botulinum toxin modifies the release of neurotransmitters that are relevant in the transduction of pain (such as CGRP, substance P and glutamate) [8,30,31]. ONA-BoNTA reduces the number of pain signals that reach the brain and consequently prevents the activation and sensitization of central neurons [30].

7. Conclusions

This article presented the primary headaches, otherwise named idiopathic, which are a large group of diseases. The etiology is unclear, and the headache is not a symptom of another known disease. The most common of these are migraine, tension-type headache and cluster headache. Many of these patients seek dental care because orofacial pain is a common presenting symptom. It would be advisable for a specialist in orofacial pain to know the criteria for the diagnosis of headaches and for headache physicians to know the semiologic aspects of orofacial pain. It is, therefore, necessary to differentiate these symptoms. Moreover, botulinum toxin would be helpful in treating bruxism or other occlusal disorders. This problem may be covered in other articles and would be helpful, especially in dental practice.

It has been well established that botulinum toxin may be an effective prophylactic treatment for chronic headache types. Botulinum toxin serotype A was originally used in neurology for the treatment of dystonia and blepharospasm. It is also widely used in the treatment of the disease of the rumen and temples of the temporomandibular muscles, as presented by Ferrillo M [32].

Currently, it is clinically used as an attractive alternative for patients with chronic migraine who do not respond positively to other drugs. ONA-BoNTA is effective in CM, not only in headache frequency and pain intensity but in other parameters, including quality of life. Recent and future developments in other headache disorders are still discussed.

However, the results of treatment are dependent on the dose, location of injection and the number of cycles.

Author Contributions: K.K. is the first and corresponding author and wrote the paper; K.K. and I.D. conceived and designed the paper, analyzed the data, contributed reagents/materials/analysis tools. All authors have read and agreed to the published version of the manuscript.

Funding: This study received no specific grant from any agency in the public, commercial or not-for profit sectors.

Institutional Review Board Statement: Not applicable.

Informed Consent Statement: Not applicable.

Data Availability Statement: Not applicable.

Conflicts of Interest: The authors declare no conflict of interest.

References

1. Headache Classification Commitee of the International Headache Society, International Classification of Headache Disorders, 3rd edition. *Cephalalgia* **2018**, *38*, 1–211. [CrossRef] [PubMed]
2. Bahra, A.; Evans, R.W. The secondary Headaches. *Cephalalgia* **2021**, *41*, 427–430. [CrossRef] [PubMed]
3. Steiner, T.J.; Stovner, L.J.; Vos, T. GBD 2015: Migraine is the third cause of disability in under 50s. *J. Headache Pain* **2016**, *17*, 104. [CrossRef] [PubMed]
4. Bigal, M.E.; Lipton, R.B. Modifiable risk factors for migraine progression. *Headache* **2006**, *46*, 1334–1343. [CrossRef] [PubMed]
5. Burch, R.C.; Buse, D.C.; Lipton, R.B. Migraine: Epidemiology, Burden and Comorbidity. *Neurol. Clin.* **2019**, *37*, 631–649. [CrossRef]
6. Aurora, S.K.; Dodick, D.W.; Turkel, C.C.; DeGryse, R.E.; Silberstein, S.D.; Lipton, R.B.; Diener, H.C.; Brin, M.F.; PREEMPT 1 Chronic Migraine Study Group. OnabotulinumtoxinA for treatment of chronic migraine: Results from the double-blind, randomized, placebo-controlled phase of the PRREMPT 1 trial. *Cephalalgia* **2010**, *30*, 793–803. [CrossRef]
7. Diener, H.C.; Dodick, D.W.; Aurora, S.K.; Turkel, C.C.; DeGryse, R.E.; Lipton, R.B.; Silberstein, S.D.; Brin, M.F.; PREEMPT 2 Chronic Migraine Study Group. OnabotulinumtoxinA for treatment of chronic migraine: Results from the double-blind, randomized, placebo-controlled phase of the PRREMPT 2 trial. *Cephalalgia* **2010**, *30*, 804–814. [CrossRef]
8. Becker, W.J. Botulinum Toxin in the Treatment of Headache. *Toxins* **2020**, *12*, 803. [CrossRef]
9. Ramachandran, R.; Yaksh, T.L. Therapeutic use of botulinum toxin in migraine: Mechanisms of action. *Br. J. Pharmacol.* **2014**, *171*, 4177–4192. [CrossRef]
10. Robertson, C.E.; Garza, I. Critical analysis of the use of onatobotulinumtoxinA (botulinum toxin type A) in migraine. *Neuropsychiatr. Dis. Treat.* **2012**, *8*, 35–48. [CrossRef]
11. Kahriman, A.; Zhu, S. Migraine and Tension-Type Headache. *Semin. Neurol.* **2018**, *38*, 608–618. [CrossRef]
12. Pihut, M.; Ferendiuk, E.; Szewczyk, M.; Kasprzyk, K.; Wieckiewicz, M. The efficiency of botulinum toxin type A for the treatment of masseter muscle pain in patients with temporomandibular joint dysfunction and tension-type headache. *J. Headache Pain* **2016**, *17*, 29. [CrossRef]
13. Ashkenazi, A.; Blumenfeld, A. OnabotulinumtoxinA for the treatment of headache. *Headache* **2013**, *53*, 54–61. [CrossRef] [PubMed]
14. Roland, S.B.; Pripp, A.H.; Msomphora, M.R.; Kvarstein, G. The efficacy of botulinum toxin A treatment for tension-type or cervivogenic headache: A systematic review and meta-analysis of randomized, placebo-controlled trials. *Scand. J. Pain* **2021**, *21*, 635–652. [CrossRef] [PubMed]
15. Gaul, C.; Holle-Lee, D.; Straube, A. Botulinum toxin type A in headache treatment: Established and experimental indications. *Nervenarzt* **2016**, *87*, 853–859. [CrossRef]
16. Lipton, R.B.; Cady, R.K.; Stewart, W.F.; Wilks, K.; Hall, C. Diagnostic lessons from the spectrum study. *Neurology* **2002**, *14*, 27–31. [CrossRef] [PubMed]
17. May, A.; Scwedt, T.J.; Magis, D.; Pozo-Rosich, P.; Evers, S.; Wang, S.J. Cluster headache. *Nat. Rev. Dis. Primers* **2018**, *1*, 18006. [CrossRef] [PubMed]
18. Hoffman, J.; May, A. Diagnosis, pathophysiology, and management of cluster headache. *Lancet Neurol.* **2018**, *17*, 75–83. [CrossRef]
19. Freund, B.; Kotchetkov, I.S.; Rao, A. The Efficacy of Botulinum Toxin in Cluster Headache: A Systematic Review. *J. Oral Facial Pain Headache* **2020**, *34*, 129–134. [CrossRef]
20. Bratbak, D.F.; Nordgard, S.; Stovner, L.J. Pilot study of sphenopalatine injection of onabotulinumtoxinA for the treatment of itractable chronic cluster headache. *Cephalalgia* **2016**, *36*, 503–509. [CrossRef]
21. Crespi, J.; Bratbak, D.; Dodick, D.W. Open-Label, Multi-Dose, Pilot Safety Study of Injection of OnabotulinumtoxinA toward the Otic Ganglion for the Treatment of Intractable Chroni Cluster Headache. *Headache* **2020**, *60*, 1632–1634. [CrossRef] [PubMed]
22. Adams, A.M.; Serrano, D.; Buse, D.C.; Reed, M.L.; Marske, V.; Fanning, K.M.; Lipton, R.B. The impact of chronic migraine: The Chronic Migraine Epidemiology and Outcomes (CaMEO) Study methods and baseline results. *Cephalalgia* **2015**, *35*, 563–578. [CrossRef] [PubMed]

23. Wang, Y.F. OnabotulinumtoxinA injection in the treatment of chronic migraine. *Prog. Brain Res.* **2020**, *255*, 171–206. [PubMed]
24. Jackson, J.; Kuriyama, A.; Hayashino, Y. Botulinum toxin A for prophylactic treatment of migraine and tension headaches in adults: A meta-analysis. *J. Am. Med. Assoc.* **2012**, *307*, 1736–1745.
25. Silberstein, S.D.; Stark, S.R.; Lucas, S.M.; Christie, S.N.; Degryse, R.E.; Turkel, C.C. Botulinum toxin type A for the prophylactic treatment of chronic daily headache: A randomized, double-blind, placebo-controlled trial. *Mayo Clin. Proc.* **2005**, *80*, 1126–1137. [CrossRef]
26. Vo, A.; Satori, R.; Jabbari, B.; Green, J.; Killgore, W.D.; Labutta, R.; Campbell, W.W. Botulinum toxin type-A in the prevention of migraine: A double-blind controlled trial. *Aviat. Space Environ. Med.* **2007**, *78*, 113–118.
27. Blumenfeld, A.; Silberstein, S.D.; Dodick, D.W.; Aurora, S.K.; Turkel, C.C.; Binder, W.J. Method of injection of onabotulinumtoxinA for chronic migraine: A safe, well-tolerated, and effective treatment paradigm based on the PREEMPT clinical program. *Headache* **2010**, *50*, 1406–1418. [CrossRef]
28. Dodick, D.W.; Mauskop, A.; Elkind, A.H.; DeGryse, R.E.; Brin, M.F.; Silberstein, S.D. Botulinum toxin type a for the prophylaxis of chronic daily headache: Subgroup analysis of patients not receiving other prophylactic medications: A randomized double-blind, placebo-cotrolled study. *Headache* **2005**, *45*, 315–324. [CrossRef]
29. Rummel, A. The long journey of botulinum neurotoxins into the synapse. *Toxicon* **2015**, *107*, 9–24. [CrossRef]
30. Burstein, R.; Blumenfeld, A.M.; Silberstein, S.D. Mechanism of Action of OnabotulinumtoxinA in Chronic Migraine: A Narrative Review. *Headache* **2020**, *60*, 1259–1272. [CrossRef]
31. Matak, I.; Lacković, Z. Botulinum toxin A, brain and pain. *Prog. Neurobiol.* **2014**, *119–120*, 39–59. [CrossRef] [PubMed]
32. Ferillo, M.; Migliaro, M.; Marotta, N.; Fortunato, F.; Bindi, M.; Pezzotti, F.; Ammendolia, A.; Giudice, A.; Foglio Bonda, P.L.; de Sira, A. Temporomandibular disorders and neck pain in primary headache patients: A retrospective machine learning study. *Acta Odontol. Scand.* **2022**, *29*, 1–7. [CrossRef] [PubMed]

toxins

MDPI

Systematic Review

Is Botulinum Toxin Effective in Treating Orofacial Neuropathic Pain Disorders? A Systematic Review

Matteo Val [1,*], Robert Delcanho [2], Marco Ferrari [1], Luca Guarda Nardini [3] and Daniele Manfredini [1]

1 Department of Biomedical Technologies, School of Dental Medicine, University of Siena, 53100 Siena, Italy
2 School of Dentistry, University of Western Australia, Perth 6009, Australia
3 Unit of Oral and Maxillofacial Surgery, Ca'Foncello Hospital, 31100 Treviso, Italy
* Correspondence: matteo.val@outlook.it

Abstract: Background: The aim of this paper is to provide a systematic review of the literature regarding the clinical use of botulinum toxin (BTX) to treat various orofacial neuropathic pain disorders (NP). Methods: A comprehensive literature search was conducted using Medline, Web of Science, and the Cochrane Library databases. Only randomized clinical trials (RCT) published between 2003 and the end of June 2023, investigating the use of BTX to treat NP, were selected. PICO guidelines were used to select and tabulate the articles. Results: A total of 6 RCTs were selected. Five articles used BTX injections to treat classical trigeminal neuralgia, and one to treat post-herpetic neuralgia. A total of 795 patients received BTX injections. The selected studies utilised different doses and methods of injections and doses. All the selected studies concluded superiority of BTX injections over placebo for reducing pain levels, and 5 out 6 of them highlighted an improvement in the patient's quality of life. Most of the studies reported transient and mild side effects. Conclusion: There is evidence of the efficacy of BTX injections in orofacial pain management. However, improved study protocols are required to provide direction for the clinical use of BTX to treat various orofacial neuropathic pain disorders.

Keywords: botulinum toxin type A; orofacial neuropathic disorders; essential trigeminal neuralgia; pain; quality of life

Key Contribution: BTX-A produces a reduction in pain levels and improvs quality of life of patients suffering from essential trigeminal neuralgia.

Citation: Val, M.; Delcanho, R.; Ferrari, M.; Guarda Nardini, L.; Manfredini, D. Is Botulinum Toxin Effective in Treating Orofacial Neuropathic Pain Disorders? A Systematic Review. *Toxins* **2023**, *15*, 541. https://doi.org/10.3390/toxins15090541

Received: 11 August 2023
Revised: 26 August 2023
Accepted: 30 August 2023
Published: 1 September 2023

1. Introduction

Pain is an unpleasant sensory and emotional experience associated with or resembling that associated with actual or potential tissue damage [1]. Specifically, neuropathic pain is caused by an injury or a disease of the somatosensory nervous system. Neuropathic pain is divided into central (pain caused by a lesion or disease of the central somatosensory nervous system) and peripheral (a disease or trauma of the peripheral somatosensory nervous system) [2].

The appropriate management of neuropathic pain can be challenging and, as with other chronic pain conditions, should be approached within a biopsychosocial framework. Pharmacological management is considered a component within an overall approach to improving patients' quality of life and function [3]. Based on systematic reviews and meta-analysis of randomized controlled clinical trials, a number of published guidelines for pharmacological treatment of neuropathic pain are available [4].

Carbamazepine and oxcarbazepine are considered first line pharmacological treatments for cranial nerve neuralgias. For other neuropathic pain disorders, to date, the highest quality evidence exists for tricyclic antidepressants, pregabalin, gabapentin, and serotonin and noradrenaline reuptake inhibitors. Tramadol, topical lidocaine, and topical capsaicin could be considered as second choices. Stronger opioids, including tapentadol, could be considered third line but are generally not considered suitable for non-cancer pain. It should be remembered that opioids and gabapentinoids have abuse potential [5].

The use of botulinum toxin type A (BTX) has gained increasing attention and importance in the management of peripheral neuropathic pain. Studies have demonstrated a moderate efficacy with reduced side effects as compared to systemically administered medication [6]. BTX is a neurotoxin derived from Clostridium botulinum and causes relaxation of skeletal muscles by inhibiting the release of acetylcholine at neuromuscular junctions [7]. BTX also has been demonstrated to inhibit the release of substance P, glutamate, and calcitonin gene-related peptide (CGRP) from sensory neurons [8]. This decreases pain perception by inhibiting both peripheral and central nervous system pain pathways [9]. A systematic review [10] showed a significant benefit of BTX injections in patients affected by neuropathic pain due to postherpetic neuralgia [11,12], spinal cord Injury [13,14], peripheral nerve lesion [15], diabetic neuropathy [16–19], post-traumatic/postoperative neuropathies [20], myofascial pain [21,22], and carpal tunnel syndrome [23]. Furthermore, numerous papers have demonstrated that BTX intervenes on the modulation of pain perception in the orofacial district [24–28]. Another study [29] highlighted the efficacy of BTX in the treatment of a patients suffering from hemifacial spasms and trigeminal neuralgia.

Although numerous studies have been published evaluating the efficacy of BTX in the management of various neuropathic pain disorders, there remains a paucity of publications specifically addressing the use of BTX for the management of orofacial neuropathic pain disorders, and any findings have not been systematically summarized. Within these premises, the aim of this paper is to systematically review the scientific evidence regarding the safety and efficacy of BTX in the management of orofacial neuropathic pain disorders which have emerged from published randomized controlled trials.

2. Materials and Methods

2.1. Search Strategy and Criteria for Selecting Articles and Registration

A systematic review of the literature addressing the use of BTX in the management of neuropathic pain affecting the orofacial area (NP) was carried out via a literature search of the MedLine and ISI Web of Sciences databases and the Cochrane Library, following the PRISMA guidelines [30]. Referenced studies within reviewed articles were also included if they met our inclusion criteria. The Pub Med database search utilized a combination of different search keywords (see Appendix A for details): botulinum toxin neuropathic pain, botulinum toxin neuropathy, botulinum toxin neuralgia, botulinum toxin burning mouth, botulinum toxin neurology, botulinum toxin glossopharyngeal neuralgia, botulinum toxin trigeminal neuralgia, botulinum toxin auriculotemporal neuralgia, botulinum toxin postherpetic, and botulinum toxin pain. This systematic review was registered, and the protocol is available on the National Institute for Health Research International prospective register of systematic reviews, PROSPERO, with the number CRD42023403119.

2.2. Inclusion Criteria

The inclusion criteria included randomized controlled clinical trials (RCTs) investigating the use of BTX to treat neuropathic pain in the orofacial region. In addition, studies had to be written in English.

2.3. Exclusion Criteria

The following publications were omitted: non-randomized controlled trials, non-controlled trials, systematic reviews or meta-analyses, non-systematic reviews, case reports, studies not reporting the use of BTX in NP, studies reporting data from previous publications, opinion papers, letters to the editor, and articles published before year 2000.

2.4. Selection of Participants

The participants included adults of both genders diagnosed with any type of neuropathic disorders/neuralgia involving the orofacial area (trigeminal neuralgia/neuropathy, auriculotemporal neuralgia/neuropathy, postherpetic neuralgia/neuropathy, nervus intermedius neuralgia/neuropathy, burning mouth syndrome, peripheral painful traumatic trigeminal neuropathy, persistent idiopathic facial pain, and central post-stroke pain) who have undergone treatment with BTX.

2.5. Methods

The review process initially addressed the titles and abstracts (TiAb screening) and then the full-text papers. Two different reviewers (MV, DM) separately performed the process and discussed the differences. The full text of the selected articles that met the eligibility criteria were retrieved and reviewed in-depth by two reviewers (RD, LGN). In each study, the following data were extracted: author (s), year of publication, study design, sample size, gender and age of participants, follow-up period, outcome variables, and results. A PICO-like [31] structured reading (i.e., BP^—patients/problem/population, BI^—intervention, BC^—comparison and BO^—outcome) was adopted, if possible, based on the following question: In patients with various NDs (P), do BTX injections (I), as compared versus other treatments (C), reduced pain levels and improve function (O)? A descriptive analysis was then conducted on the selected studies. As the timeline in which the articles were selected was very wide, it was impossible to structure the review according to PICOT (in which T stands for "time frame").

2.6. Statistical Analysis

The intent was to perform a meta-analysis for this systematic review; however, due to the marked heterogeneity of the studies, this proved impossible. A descriptive analysis of the studies was performed.

2.7. Quality of RCT Selected

Grading of the level of evidence was based on the work of Sackett and colleagues and is summarized in Figure 1 [32]. The Jadad score (Figure 2) was used to assess the quality of the double blinding, randomization, and flow of patients. The scores ranged from 0 (bad) to 5 (good). Based on these, the overall quality of the methods was assessed.

Level	Intervention (Group) studies
I	Systematic review of randomized controlled trials (RCTs) Large RCT (with narrow confidence intervals) (n >100)
II	Smaller RCT's (with wider confidence intervals) (n<100) Systematic reviews of cohort studies "Outcomes research" (very large ecologic studies)
III	Cohort studies (must have concurrent control group) Systematic reviews of case control studies
IV	Case series Cohort study without concurrent control group (e.g. with historical control group) Case-control Study
V	Expert Opinion Case study or report Bench research Expert opinion based on theory or physiologic research Common sense/anecdotes

Figure 1. Grading of the level of evidence is based on the work of Sackett and colleagues.

Item	Maximum point	Description
Randomization	2	1 point if randomization is mentioned 1 additional point if the method of randomization is appropriate Deduct 1 point if the method of randomization is inappropriate (minimum 0)
Blinding	2	1 point if blinding is mentioned 1 additional point if the method of blinding is appropriate Deduct 1 point if the method of blinding is inappropriate (minimum 0)
An account of all patients	1	The fate of all patients in the trial is known. If there are no data the reason is stated

Figure 2. Jadad Scale.

2.8. *Outcome*

Primary Outcomes of the reviewed studies were:

- Pain levels were evaluated using a reliable, validated scale, like the visual analogue scale (VAS);
- If a validated tool was available, health-related quality of life was assessed;
- The percentage of participants who experienced major adverse events were measured, including life-threatening situations, hospitalization, or incidents that caused serious disability or incapacity (e.g., infection, dysphagia);
- Participants with at least 1 adverse event (e.g., hypersensitivity reactions such as anaphylaxis, urticaria, soft tissue oedema, dyspnea, or allergic reaction) were evaluated.

Secondary Outcomes were:

- Function was assessed by a validated questionnaire;
- Utilisation of analgesic medication was assessed by type and dose used per day.

3. Results

A total of 795 papers were found. Six (n = 6) randomized clinical trials were selected via the keywords searched (see Appendix A). The flowcharts of the article selection process for all the search queries can be found in Figure 3. Due to the wide variability in the study methods and the evaluation of results, a meta-analysis of findings could not be performed. Furthermore, despite the search with specific keywords for orofacial neuropathic pain disorders, the only RCTs that were found were for treatment with botulinum toxin for classical trigeminal neuralgia [33–37] and post herpetic neuralgia [12]. Finally, the psychological aspect of pain perception holds significant value and can potentially impact the study's results, but none of the studies assessed the psychological condition in the patient's selection process.

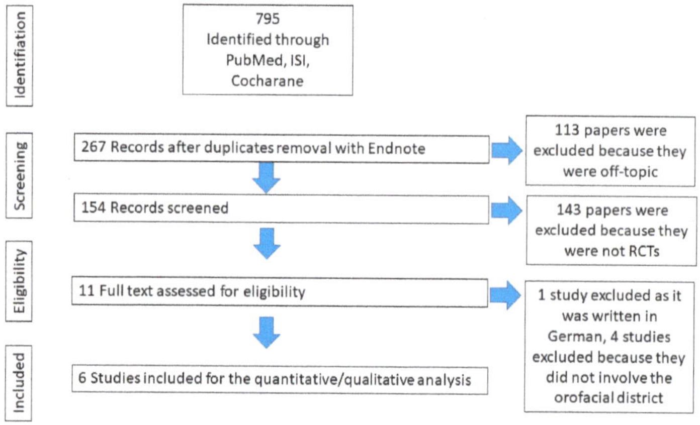

Figure 3. Flowchart that highlights the process of article selection.

3.1. *Study Characteristics*

Table 1 displays the characteristics of the included studies (published between 2003 and 2023).

They included a total of seven RCTs (n = 365 patients) of whom 226 were treated with the injection of BTX. Males outnumbered females (M:F = 192:173). The mean age for both case and control groups ranged between 46.4 (±7.7) and 77.73 (±8.41). There was no significant difference between BTX-A and the control groups in terms of frequency of attacks and pain severity before treatment. All selected studies had a placebo (saline injection) control group with the exception of Zhang et al. (2017) [34]. Zhang et al. (2014) [33] compared two groups of patients suffering from trigeminal neuralgia treated with different doses of BTX (25 U BTX group and 75 U BTX group) against a placebo. A later study [34] compared a single dose versus a repeat dose. The single dose group received a first dose of 70–100 U with the second group receiving an initial dose of 50–70 units, which was repeated two weeks later. Finally, Xiao et al. [12] was the only paper that compared BTX with another injected medication (lidocaine) in addition to the placebo group.

3.2. *Quality of RCTs Selected*

Table 2 shows the Jadad score and the level of evidence of the six selected items. The level of evidence is considered high, as all studies are randomized controlled trials (RCTs). However, the study conducted by Zhang et al. (2017) [34], which involved 100 participants, had low quality in terms of double blinding, randomization, and patient flow. On the other hand, Shehata et al. [36], Wu et al. [38], and Xiao et al. [12] had good Jadad scores.

3.3. *Types, Number of Administrations, Sites and Doses of Botulinum Toxin, and Side-Effects*

All studies [12,33–37] evaluated the effectiveness of botulinum toxin type A, and the sites of injection were selected on the basis of subjective pain perception and areas demonstrating evidence of tactile allodynia. The amount of BTX-A injected, injection technique, the site, and the number of injections varied between the studies. The amount of BTX-A injected ranged from a minimum of 25 U to a maximum of 140 U) [34]. The number of injection sites ranged from 8 [36] to 25 [33] depending on the width of the interested area. In each study, the injections were performed at a distance of 10–15 mm from each other. Most of the studies reported transient and mild side effects. The reported side effects were facial asymmetry, weakness, hematoma, oedema at the site of injection, itching, and pain at the site of injection [12,33,34,36,37]. Zuniga and colleagues noted that one participant in the BTX group and five participants in the placebo group experienced hiccups or anaesthesia in the affected area [35]. In addition, three individuals from the BTX group and three patients from the placebo group exhibited a decrease in the corneal reflex.

Table 1. Characteristics of the studies related to the interventions.

Study	Year	Diagnosis	Sample Size (Test/Control)	Test/Control	Site of Injection	Repeated Injection	Weeks between First and Second Injection	Follow-Up	Drop-Out
Shehata [36]	2013	Trigeminal Neuralgia	20 (BTX 10: saline10)	BTX-A (Botox®) (100 U Botox in 2 mL preservative-free normal saline, resulting in a concentration of 5 units/0.1 mL) or placebo (2 mL 0.9% NaCl).	"follow the pain" method. If the branch of the mandible is affected, a higher amount of toxin is injected at the back of the masseter muscle to prevent any unwanted cosmetic outcomes.	No	0	12 weeks	0
Wu [37]	2012	Trigeminal Neuralgia	42 (BTX 22: saline 20)	intradermal and/or submucosal injection of BTX-A (75 U/1.5 mL;) or saline (1.5 mL)	"follow the pain" method.	No	0	12 weeks	2
Xiao [12]	2010	Postherpetic neuralgia	60 (20:20:20)	The lidocaine group (0.5% lidocaine) acted as an active control. Non-preserved saline (0.9%) was used for the placebo group. For the BTX-A group, aliquots of 100 IU/vial of BTX-A were reconstituted with 20 mL of saline solution.	Subjects received subcutaneous injections into the affected area, specifically the area demonstrating evidence of tactile allodynia.	No	0	3 months	4
Zhang [34]	2017	Trigeminal Neuralgia	100 (50:50)	Patients in the single-dose group received a local BTX-A injection of 70 to 100 U. The repeated-dose group received an initial BTX-A injection of 50 to 70 U and then another of equal volume 2 weeks later.	"follow the pain" method	Yes	2 weeks	6 months	19
Zhang [33]	2014	Trigeminal Neuralgia	84 placebo (n = 28); BTX-A 25 U (n = 27); BTX-A 75 U (n = 29)	Each vial contained either active botulinum toxin type A (25 U or 75 U) or matching placebo. All three vials were identical in appearance and were reconstituted with 1 mL saline solution (0.9%). For treatment, 1 mL was drawn from vials, and the injections were administered intradermally and/or submucosally.	"follow the pain" method	No	0	8 weeks	0
Zúñiga [35]	2013	Trigeminal Neuralgia	36 (BTX 20: saline 16)	1 mL 0.9% saline plus 50 U of BTX or only 1 mL of 0.9% saline injected subcutaneously in the affected area.	Among the path of the branch/branches involved, patients with involvement of the third branch of the trigeminal nerve also received intramuscularly either 10 U of BTX or matching placebo in the masseter muscle, ipsilateral to the pain location.	No	0	3 months	5

Table 2. Jadad score and the level of evidence of the 8 selected items.

Study	Year	Type of Study	Level of Evidence	Jadad Score
Shehata [36]	2013	RCT double blind	II	5
Wu [37]	2012	RCT double blind	II	4
Xiao [12]	2010	RCT double blind	II	4
Zhang [34]	2017	RCT	I	2
Zhang [33]	2014	RCT double blind	II	2
Zúñiga [35]	2013	RCT double blind	II	3

3.4. Period of Follow-Up and Quality of Life and Pain Assessments

The longest period of follow-up was 6 months) [34] while the shortest follow-up time was 8 weeks) [33]. There was lack of homogeneity in the choice of quality of life assessment questionnaires in the various studies. Zhang et al. in 2014 [33] evaluated the overall response to treatment based on the Patient Global Impression of Change (PGIC) scale but did not evaluate the improvement in quality of life in his later study. Other quality of life assessment strategies utilized were the [35] Short Form (36) (SF36) [35] and 10-point quality of life (QoL) scale adopted from the American Chronic Pain Association [36],and sleeping time (hours), daily activity, diet, and stance in a day [12].

3.5. Effect on Pain Reduction

All the studies selected [12,33–37] used the visual analogue scale (VAS) to evaluate pain.

All studies included in the review demonstrated a statistically significant effect of BTX injections reducing pain intensity compared to placebo. The onset of analgesic effects averaged between 7 [12,33] and 15 [36,37] days, lasting up to 3 months [12,35]. Studies comparing different doses of BTX failed to demonstrate a significant difference in pain relief at higher doses. Table 3 summarizes the results obtained in pain management.

Table 3. Summary of the effect of BTX in pain management.

Study	Year	Results in Pain Management
Shehata [36]	2013	Pain reduction at the 12-week endpoint was significant in the BTX group ($p < 0.0001$). The BTX-A group showed a decrease in VAS scores starting from week 2 and maintained it throughout the follow-up period. Furthermore, a significant reduction in paroxysm frequency was observed in the BTX-A group compared to the placebo group from week 2 onwards ($p < 0.0001$).
Wu [37]	2012	At week 2, BTX-A showed a significant decrease in the average VAS scores compared to the placebo. The results showed that BTX-A was significantly better than the placebo in reducing the frequency of attacks. This effect was noticeable as early as the first week.
Xiao [12]	2010	The VAS pain scores decreased in all three groups at day 7 and 3 months after treatment ($p < 0.01$). The group that received BTX-A had a greater decrease in VAS pain scores compared to the lidocaine and placebo groups, which was more significant at day 7 and 3 months after treatment ($p < 0.01$). Out of the three groups tested, the BTX-A group had the lowest percentage (21.1%) of subjects using opioids after treatment, compared to the lidocaine (52.6%) and placebo (66.7%) groups. This difference was statistically significant ($p < 0.01$).
Zhang [34]	2017	The group that received a single dose of the drug had a noticeably longer effect time ($p = 0.032$). The drug response rates between the single-dose and repeated-dose groups did not show significant differences ($p > 0.05$).

Table 3. *Cont.*

Study	Year	Results in Pain Management
Zhang [33]	2014	During the study, the groups that received doses of 25 U and 75 U experienced a significant reduction in VAS scores compared to the placebo group as early as week 1. Throughout the study, there was no significant difference in VAS scores between the 25 U and 75 U groups. At week 8, the response rates for the 25 U group (70.4%) and 75 U group (86.2%) were significantly higher than the response rate for the placebo group (32.1%). However, there was no significant difference in response rates between the 25 U and 75 U groups.
Zúñiga [35]	2013	After three months of the injection, a noticeable contrast was detected in the average VAS score between individuals who received BTX treatment and those who received placebo treatment (VAS 4.75 vs. 6.94, respectively; *t*-test, $p = 0.01$).

3.6. Quality of Life

Most of all the selected works [12,33,34,36,37], despite using different methods, demonstrated improved quality of life of for patients treated with BTX.

In the management of trigeminal neuralgia, Shehata et al. [36] showed a significant decrease in the number of weekly rescue medications and an increase in the QoL functioning scale following BTX injections. Two studies utilizing the PGIC found that patients who received BTX had a "great improvement" or "very much improvement" in pain symptoms compared with the placebo group ($p < 0.01$ in both studies). Moreover, Zhang et al. (2014) [33] failed to find a significant difference between lower and higher BTX doses (25 U and 75 U) in the improvement of PGIC scores ($p > 0.05$). However, using the SF36, Zuniga et al. [35] failed to find an improvement in quality of life following BTX administration.

Xiao et al. [12] recorded sleep time (hours) to assess any improvement in the quality of life of patients suffering from post-herpetic neuralgia. Over the course of three months post-treatment, the amount of time each group slept consistently increased from day one ($p < 0.01$). The amount of time spent sleeping was significantly increased with the use of BTX-A if compared with the other two group (injected with lidocaine and placebo) ($p < 0.01$).

4. Discussion

The treatment of neuropathies/neuralgias in the orofacial region represents a clinical challenge for both patients and health care providers. Orally administered medications (and in particular carbamazepine for trigeminal neuralgia) are considered the gold standard in the treatment of NP; however, these medications can be poorly tolerated and associated with severe side effects. Surgical therapies such as microvascular decompression are invasive and with associated morbidity and even mortality. If an alternative, efficacious treatment with reduced side effects could be established, the treating practitioner will have further management options at their disposal. BTX seems to have these characteristics, and, since 2002 [29], it has been used successfully in the management of trigeminal neuralgia [8,9]. The ability of BTX in reducing pain perception in other orofacial pathologies has been widely demonstrated [24–28].

Unfortunately, using our strict inclusion criteria to analyse the literature, only two orofacial neuropathic pain conditions were identified: classical trigeminal neuralgia [33–37] and post-herpetic neuralgia [12]. Publications addressing the use of BTX to treat other likely orofacial neuropathic pain conditions such as burning mouth disorder, post traumatic trigeminal neuropathic pain, persistent idiopathic facial, and dentoalveolar pain simply failed to meet the criteria used for inclusion in this review. There is also low-quality evidence for use of BTX injections to treat some conditions possibly related to trigeminal neuralgia, such as SUNCT and SUNA. It is evident that additional research, beyond just case reports, is necessary to establish high-quality evidence on the effectiveness of using BTX to treat the aforementioned conditions, as such evidence is currently non-existent. The use of BTX in these situations is therefore lacking a solid scientific evidence base but could be considered clinically on an 'ad hoc' basis perhaps where other treatments have failed.

The studies that were included had small sample sizes, with only three out of six studies being carried out with more than 50 participants [12,33,34]. The high cost of botulinum toxin and the fact that the management of neuropathic disorders with BTX is "off-label" may explain the low number of studies and participants. All the studies stated the diagnostic criteria used for the different disorders.

Furthermore, all patients in the selected studies had been treated with anti-epileptic medications (usually carbamazepine or oxcarbazepine, with gabapentin being the next most popular), which were all maintained during the studies. Details of the medications being taken were provided in the studies. However, Xiao et al. [12] suspended all medications and introduced transcutaneous electrical nerve stimulation (TENS) in the management of pain during the trial.

The sites of BTX injections varied between the different articles, with some being directly into trigger zones [33–37] and others within the affected dermatomes/oral mucosa involved [12]. BTX was injected intradermally [33,34,37], submucosally [33,34] or subcutaneously[12,35,36], but the depth of injection in millimetres was never stated.

The paper which compared single different dosages of BTX [33] and a second dose two weeks later [34] found no statistical difference in VAS scores where a higher dose of BTX was used. Higher doses were found to be safe.

All the studies demonstrated that BTX had a statistically significant efficacy in pain management compared to placebo [12,33,35–37] and lidocaine [12]. Furthermore, all the papers included in this review stated that the different indices for quality of life assessment are significantly improved compared to placebo. Due to these findings and the fact that each study utilised different dosages from very low (25 U [33]) to very high (140 U [34]), it was not possible to identify a common or recommended protocol for the management of orofacial neuralgia with botulinum toxin. It is unclear from the included studies which patients may best benefit from using BTX injections. There is weak evidence that BTX further reduces pain intensity when used as an adjunct to the commonly used anti-epileptic drugs [39].

BTX could prove to be exceptionally beneficial for elderly patients who are unable to bear the adverse effects of medication and may not be apt for, or apprehensive of, severe complications from microvascular decompression surgery [38]. It may have use as a "rescue" strategy for acute exacerbations of primary trigeminal neuralgia [40]. In doses of 100–300 U, there is evidence of BTX efficacy to treat localized peripheral neuropathic pain. This may be particularly helpful for patients who exhibit allodynia, limited thermal deficit, and have residual intraepidermal nerve fibres as determined by a skin punch biopsy [14,41].

The evidence from this systematic review suggests that botulinum toxin type A (BTX-A), when compared to placebo, probably has a clinically significant benefit in the treatment of the orofacial neuropathic pain disorders, trigeminal neuralgia, and post herpetic neuralgia. The overall outcomes consistently favoured BTX-A compared with placebo across studies, while also considering that systemic side effects were minimal and transient. It should be noted that different diagnostic criteria were used for patient selection (tIHS [36], ICHD-2 [33,34,37] and the classification of chronic pain [35]) and the differences between the infiltration protocols do not make these studies directly comparable.

5. Conclusions

Previous reviews of the literature [24,42] have demonstrated evidence of the efficacy of BTX injections in pain management. However, in order to provide a protocol for the tailored use of BTX to treat different orofacial neuropathic pain conditions, improved study protocols, e.g., patient selection, phenotyping, injection techniques, dosing, intervals between doses, etc., and an increased homogeneity of research protocols are required. Furthermore, studies utilizing BTX to treat other presumed orofacial neuropathic conditions are required before recommendations for routine clinical use can be made.

Author Contributions: Conceptualization, M.V. and D.M.; methodology, D.M.; validation, D.M., L.G.N. and M.V.; formal analysis, R.D.; data curation, M.V. and M.F.; writing—original draft preparation, M.V.; writing—review and editing, R.D., D.M. and M.F.; visualization, M.F.; supervision, L.G.N. All authors have read and agreed to the published version of the manuscript.

Funding: This research received no external funding.

Institutional Review Board Statement: Not applicable.

Informed Consent Statement: Not applicable.

Data Availability Statement: No new data were created in this study. Data sharing is not applicable to this article.

Conflicts of Interest: The authors declare no conflict of interest.

Appendix A

Full list of combination of keywords:

(("botulinum toxins"[MeSH Terms] OR ("botulinum"[All Fields] AND "toxins"[All Fields]) OR "botulinum toxins"[All Fields] OR ("botulinum"[All Fields] AND "toxin"[All Fields]) OR "botulinum toxin"[All Fields]) AND ("neuralgia"[MeSH Terms] OR "neuralgia"[All Fields] OR ("neuropathic"[All Fields] AND "pain"[All Fields]) OR "neuropathic pain"[All Fields])).

(("botulinum toxins"[MeSH Terms] OR ("botulinum"[All Fields] AND "toxins"[All Fields]) OR "botulinum toxins"[All Fields] OR ("botulinum"[All Fields] AND "toxin"[All Fields]) OR "botulinum toxin"[All Fields]) AND ("neuropathies"[All Fields] OR "neuropathy"[All Fields])).

(("botulinum toxins"[MeSH Terms] OR ("botulinum"[All Fields] AND "toxins"[All Fields]) OR "botulinum toxins"[All Fields] OR ("botulinum"[All Fields] AND "toxin"[All Fields]) OR "botulinum toxin"[All Fields]) AND ("neuralgia"[MeSH Terms] OR "neuralgia"[All Fields] OR "neuralgias"[All Fields]))

(("botulinum toxins"[MeSH Terms] OR ("botulinum"[All Fields] AND "toxins"[All Fields]) OR "botulinum toxins"[All Fields] OR ("botulinum"[All Fields] AND "toxin"[All Fields]) OR "botulinum toxin"[All Fields]) AND ("burning"[All Fields] OR "burns"[MeSH Terms] OR "burns"[All Fields] OR "burned"[All Fields] OR "burnings"[All Fields]) AND ("mouth"[MeSH Terms] OR "mouth"[All Fields] OR "mouths"[All Fields] OR "mouth s"[All Fields] OR "mouthed"[All Fields] OR "mouthful"[All Fields] OR "mouthfuls"[All Fields] OR "mouthing"[All Fields]) AND ("syndrom"[All Fields] OR "syndromal"[All Fields] OR "syndromally"[All Fields] OR "syndrome"[MeSH Terms] OR "syndrome"[All Fields] OR "syndromes"[All Fields] OR "syndrome s"[All Fields] OR "syndromic"[All Fields] OR "syndroms"[All Fields]))

(("botulinum toxins"[MeSH Terms] OR ("botulinum"[All Fields] AND "toxins"[All Fields]) OR "botulinum toxins"[All Fields] OR ("botulinum"[All Fields] AND "toxin"[All Fields]) OR "botulinum toxin"[All Fields]) AND ("neurology"[MeSH Terms] OR "neurology"[All Fields] OR "neurology s"[All Fields]))

(("botulinum toxins"[MeSH Terms] OR ("botulinum"[All Fields] AND "toxins"[All Fields]) OR "botulinum toxins"[All Fields] OR ("botulinum"[All Fields] AND "toxin"[All Fields]) OR "botulinum toxin"[All Fields]) AND "glossopharingeal"[All Fields] AND ("neuralgia"[MeSH Terms] OR "neuralgia"[All Fields] OR "neuralgias"[All Fields]))

(("botulinum toxins"[MeSH Terms] OR ("botulinum"[All Fields] AND "toxins"[All Fields]) OR "botulinum toxins"[All Fields] OR ("botulinum"[All Fields] AND "toxin"[All Fields]) OR "botulinum toxin"[All Fields]) AND ("trigeminal neuralgia"[MeSH Terms] OR ("trigeminal"[All Fields] AND "neuralgia"[All Fields]) OR "trigeminal neuralgia"[All Fields]))

(("botulinum toxins"[MeSH Terms] OR ("botulinum"[All Fields] AND "toxins"[All Fields]) OR "botulinum toxins"[All Fields] OR ("botulinum"[All Fields] AND "toxin"[All

Fields]) OR "botulinum toxin"[All Fields]) AND "auriculotemporal"[All Fields] AND ("neuralgia"[MeSH Terms] OR "neuralgia"[All Fields] OR "neuralgias"[All Fields]))

(("botulinum toxins"[MeSH Terms] OR ("botulinum"[All Fields] AND "toxins"[All Fields]) OR "botulinum toxins"[All Fields] OR ("botulinum"[All Fields] AND "toxin"[All Fields]) OR "botulinum toxin"[All Fields]) AND "postherpetic"[All Fields])

(("botulinum toxins"[MeSH Terms] OR ("botulinum"[All Fields] AND "toxins"[All Fields]) OR "botulinum toxins"[All Fields] OR ("botulinum"[All Fields] AND "toxin"[All Fields]) OR "botulinum toxin"[All Fields]) AND ("pain"[MeSH Terms] OR "pain"[All Fields]))

(("botulinum toxins"[MeSH Terms] OR ("botulinum"[All Fields] AND "toxins"[All Fields]) OR "botulinum toxins"[All Fields] OR ("botulinum"[All Fields] AND "toxin"[All Fields]) OR "botulinum toxin"[All Fields]) AND ("neuralgia"[MeSH Terms] OR "neuralgia"[All Fields] OR ("neuropathic"[All Fields] AND "pain"[All Fields]) OR "neuropathic pain"[All Fields]) AND "After"[All Fields] AND ("neck dissection"[MeSH Terms] OR ("neck"[All Fields] AND "dissection"[All Fields]) OR "neck dissection"[All Fields]))

(("botulinum toxins"[MeSH Terms] OR ("botulinum"[All Fields] AND "toxins"[All Fields]) OR "botulinum toxins"[All Fields] OR ("botulinum"[All Fields] AND "toxin"[All Fields]) OR "botulinum toxin"[All Fields]) AND ("pain"[MeSH Terms] OR "pain"[All Fields]) AND ("surgery"[MeSH Subheading] OR "surgery"[All Fields] OR "surgical procedures, operative"[MeSH Terms] OR ("surgical"[All Fields] AND "procedures"[All Fields] AND "operative"[All Fields]) OR "operative surgical procedures"[All Fields] OR "general surgery"[MeSH Terms] OR ("general"[All Fields] AND "surgery"[All Fields]) OR "general surgery"[All Fields] OR "surgery s"[All Fields] OR "surgerys"[All Fields] OR "surgeries"[All Fields]))

References

1. Raja, S.N.; Carr, D.B.; Cohen, M.; Finnerup, N.B.; Flor, H.; Gibson, S.; Keefe, F.J.; Mogil, J.S.; Ringkamp, M.; Sluka, K.A.; et al. The revised International Association for the Study of Pain definition of pain: Concepts, challenges, and compromises. *Pain* **2020**, *161*, 1976–1982. [CrossRef]
2. Headache Classification Committee of the International Headache Society (IHS). The International Classification of Headache Disorders, 3rd edition. *Cephalalgia Int. J. Headache* **2018**, *38*, 1–211. [CrossRef] [PubMed]
3. Murnion, B.P. Neuropathic pain: Current definition and review of drug treatment. *Aust. Prescr.* **2018**, *41*, 60–63. [CrossRef] [PubMed]
4. Finnerup, N.B.; Attal, N.; Haroutounian, S.; McNicol, E.; Baron, R.; Dworkin, R.H.; Gilron, I.; Haanpää, M.; Hansson, P.; Jensen, T.S.; et al. Pharmacotherapy for neuropathic pain in adults: A systematic review and meta-analysis. *Lancet Neurol.* **2015**, *14*, 162–173. [CrossRef] [PubMed]
5. Attal, N. Pharmacological treatments of neuropathic pain: The latest recommendations. *Rev. Neurol.* **2019**, *175*, 46–50. [CrossRef] [PubMed]
6. Lakra, C.; Cohen, H. A clinical review of the use of Botulinum Toxin type A in managing central neuropathic pain in patients with spinal cord injury. *J. Spinal Cord Med.* **2022**, *45*, 651–655. [CrossRef]
7. Pearce, L.B.; First, E.R.; MacCallum, R.D.; Gupta, A. Pharmacologic characterization of botulinum toxin for basic science and medicine. *Toxicon Off. J. Int. Soc. Toxinology* **1997**, *35*, 1373–1412. [CrossRef]
8. Lucioni, A.; Bales, G.T.; Lotan, T.L.; McGehee, D.S.; Cook, S.P.; Rapp, D.E. Botulinum toxin type A inhibits sensory neuropeptide release in rat bladder models of acute injury and chronic inflammation. *BJU Int.* **2008**, *101*, 366–370. [CrossRef]
9. Aoki, K.R. Review of a proposed mechanism for the antinociceptive action of botulinum toxin type A. *Neurotoxicology* **2005**, *26*, 785–793. [CrossRef]
10. Lippi, L.; de Sire, A.; Folli, A.; D'Abrosca, F.; Grana, E.; Baricich, A.; Carda, S.; Invernizzi, M. Multidimensional Effectiveness of Botulinum Toxin in Neuropathic Pain: A Systematic Review of Randomized Clinical Trials. *Toxins* **2022**, *14*, 308. [CrossRef]
11. Apalla, Z.; Sotiriou, E.; Lallas, A.; Lazaridou, E.; Ioannides, D. Botulinum toxin A in postherpetic neuralgia: A parallel, randomized, double-blind, single-dose, placebo-controlled trial. *Clin. J. Pain* **2013**, *29*, 857–864. [CrossRef] [PubMed]
12. Xiao, L.; Mackey, S.; Hui, H.; Xong, D.; Zhang, Q.; Zhang, D. Subcutaneous injection of botulinum toxin a is beneficial in postherpetic neuralgia. *Pain Med.* **2010**, *11*, 1827–1833. [CrossRef] [PubMed]
13. Chun, A.; Levy, I.; Yang, A.; Delgado, A.; Tsai, C.Y.; Leung, E.; Taylor, K.; Kolakowsky-Hayner, S.; Huang, V.; Escalon, M.; et al. Treatment of at-level spinal cord injury pain with botulinum toxin A. *Spinal Cord Ser. Cases* **2019**, *5*, 77. [CrossRef] [PubMed]
14. Han, Z.A.; Song, D.H.; Oh, H.M.; Chung, M.E. Botulinum toxin type A for neuropathic pain in patients with spinal cord injury. *Ann. Neurol.* **2016**, *79*, 569–578. [CrossRef]

15. Attal, N.; de Andrade, D.C.; Adam, F.; Ranoux, D.; Teixeira, M.J.; Galhardoni, R.; Raicher, I.; Üçeyler, N.; Sommer, C.; Bouhassira, D. Safety and efficacy of repeated injections of botulinum toxin A in peripheral neuropathic pain (BOTNEP): A randomised, double-blind, placebo-controlled trial. *Lancet Neurol.* **2016**, *15*, 555–565. [CrossRef]
16. Ghasemi, M.; Ansari, M.; Basiri, K.; Shaigannejad, V. The effects of intradermal botulinum toxin type a injections on pain symptoms of patients with diabetic neuropathy. *J. Res. Med. Sci.* **2014**, *19*, 106–111.
17. Salehi, H.; Moussaei, M.; Kamiab, Z.; Vakilian, A. The effects of botulinum toxin type A injection on pain symptoms, quality of life, and sleep quality of patients with diabetic neuropathy: A randomized double-blind clinical trial. *Iran J. Neurol.* **2019**, *18*, 99–107.
18. Taheri, M.; Sedaghat, M.; Solhpour, A.; Rostami, P.; Safarpour Lima, B. The Effect of Intradermal Botulinum Toxin a injections on painful diabetic polyneuropathy. *Diabetes Metab. Syndr.* **2020**, *14*, 1823–1828. [CrossRef]
19. Yuan, R.Y.; Sheu, J.J.; Yu, J.M.; Chen, W.T.; Tseng, I.J.; Chang, H.H.; Hu, C.J. Botulinum toxin for diabetic neuropathic pain: A randomized double-blind crossover trial. *Neurology* **2009**, *72*, 1473–1478. [CrossRef]
20. Ranoux, D.; Attal, N.; Morain, F.; Bouhassira, D. Botulinum toxin type A induces direct analgesic effects in chronic neuropathic pain. *Ann. Neurol.* **2008**, *64*, 274–283. [CrossRef]
21. Lee, H.J.; Lee, J.H.; Yi, K.H.; Kim, H.J. Anatomical analysis of the motor endplate zones of the suprascapular nerve to the infraspinatus muscle and its clinical significance in managing pain disorder. *J. Anat.* **2023**, *243*, 467–474. [CrossRef] [PubMed]
22. Yi, K.H.; Lee, K.L.; Lee, J.H.; Hu, H.W.; Kim, H.J. Guidance to trigger point injection for treating myofascial pain syndrome: Intramuscular neural distribution of the quadratus lumborum. *Clin. Anat.* **2022**, *35*, 1100–1106. [CrossRef] [PubMed]
23. Breuer, B.; Sperber, K.; Wallenstein, S.; Kiprovski, K.; Calapa, A.; Snow, B.; Pappagallo, M. Clinically significant placebo analgesic response in a pilot trial of botulinum B in patients with hand pain and carpal tunnel syndrome. *Pain Med.* **2006**, *7*, 16–24. [CrossRef] [PubMed]
24. Delcanho, R.; Val, M.; Guarda Nardini, L.; Manfredini, D. Botulinum Toxin for Treating Temporomandibular Disorders: What is the Evidence? *J. Oral Facial Pain Headache* **2022**, *36*, 6–20. [CrossRef] [PubMed]
25. Guarda-Nardini, L.; Manfredini, D.; Salamone, M.; Salmaso, L.; Tonello, S.; Ferronato, G. Efficacy of botulinum toxin in treating myofascial pain in bruxers: A controlled placebo pilot study. *Cranio J. Craniomandib. Pract.* **2008**, *26*, 126–135. [CrossRef]
26. Guarda-Nardini, L.; Stecco, A.; Stecco, C.; Masiero, S.; Manfredini, D. Myofascial pain of the jaw muscles: Comparison of short-term effectiveness of botulinum toxin injections and fascial manipulation technique. *Cranio J. Craniomandib. Pract.* **2012**, *30*, 95–102. [CrossRef]
27. De la Torre Canales, G.; Poluha, R.L.; Alvarez Pinzón, Y.N.; Rodrigues Conti, P.C.; Manfredini, D.; Sánchez-Ayala, A.; Rizzatti-Barbosa, C.M. Effects of Botulinum Toxin Type A on the Psychosocial Features of Myofascial Pain TMD Subjects: A Randomized Controlled Trial. *J. Oral Facial Pain Headache* **2021**, *35*, 288–296. [CrossRef]
28. De la Torre Canales, G.; Alvarez-Pinzon, N.; Muñoz-Lora, V.R.M.; Vieira Peroni, L.; Farias Gomes, A.; Sánchez-Ayala, A.; Haiter-Neto, F.; Manfredini, D.; Rizzatti-Barbosa, C.M. Efficacy and Safety of Botulinum Toxin Type A on Persistent Myofascial Pain: A Randomized Clinical Trial. *Toxins* **2020**, *12*, 395. [CrossRef]
29. Micheli, F.; Scorticati, M.C.; Raina, G. Beneficial effects of botulinum toxin type a for patients with painful tic convulsif. *Clin. Neuropharmacol.* **2002**, *25*, 260–262. [CrossRef]
30. Page, M.J.; McKenzie, J.E.; Bossuyt, P.M.; Boutron, I.; Hoffmann, T.C.; Mulrow, C.D.; Shamseer, L.; Tetzlaff, J.M.; Akl, E.A.; Brennan, S.E.; et al. The PRISMA 2020 statement: An updated guideline for reporting systematic reviews. *Syst Rev* **2021**, *10*, 89. [CrossRef]
31. Moher, D.; Liberati, A.; Tetzlaff, J.; Altman, D.G. Preferred reporting items for systematic reviews and meta-analyses: The PRISMA statement. *J. Clin. Epidemiol.* **2009**, *62*, 1006–1012. [CrossRef] [PubMed]
32. Richardson, P.E. David Sackett and the birth of Evidence Based Medicine: How to Practice and Teach EBM. *BMJ* **2015**, *350*, h3089. [CrossRef] [PubMed]
33. Zhang, H.; Lian, Y.; Ma, Y.; Chen, Y.; He, C.; Xie, N.; Wu, C. Two doses of botulinum toxin type A for the treatment of trigeminal neuralgia: Observation of therapeutic effect from a randomized, double-blind, placebo-controlled trial. *J. Headache Pain* **2014**, *15*, 65. [CrossRef] [PubMed]
34. Zhang, H.; Lian, Y.; Xie, N.; Chen, C.; Zheng, Y. Single-dose botulinum toxin type a compared with repeated-dose for treatment of trigeminal neuralgia: A pilot study. *J. Headache Pain* **2017**, *18*, 81. [CrossRef] [PubMed]
35. Zúñiga, C.; Piedimonte, F.; Díaz, S.; Micheli, F. Acute treatment of trigeminal neuralgia with onabotulinum toxin A. *Clin. Neuropharmacol.* **2013**, *36*, 146–150. [CrossRef]
36. Shehata, H.S.; El-Tamawy, M.S.; Shalaby, N.M.; Ramzy, G. Botulinum toxin-type A: Could it be an effective treatment option in intractable trigeminal neuralgia? *J. Headache Pain* **2013**, *14*, 92. [CrossRef]
37. Wu, C.J.; Lian, Y.J.; Zheng, Y.K.; Zhang, H.F.; Chen, Y.; Xie, N.C.; Wang, L.J. Botulinum toxin type A for the treatment of trigeminal neuralgia: Results from a randomized, double-blind, placebo-controlled trial. *Cephalalgia Int. J. Headache* **2012**, *32*, 443–450. [CrossRef]
38. Wu, S.; Lian, Y.; Zhang, H.; Chen, Y.; Wu, C.; Li, S.; Zheng, Y.; Wang, Y.; Cheng, W.; Huang, Z. Botulinum Toxin Type A for refractory trigeminal neuralgia in older patients: A better therapeutic effect. *J. Pain Res.* **2019**, *12*, 2177–2186. [CrossRef]
39. Chong, M.S.; Bahra, A.; Zakrzewska, J.M. Guidelines for the management of trigeminal neuralgia. *Cleve. Clin. J. Med.* **2023**, *90*, 355–362. [CrossRef]

40. Moore, D.; Chong, M.S.; Shetty, A.; Zakrzewska, J.M. A systematic review of rescue analgesic strategies in acute exacerbations of primary trigeminal neuralgia. *Br. J. Anaesth.* **2019**, *123*, e385–e396. [CrossRef]
41. Moisset, X.; Bouhassira, D.; Avez Couturier, J.; Alchaar, H.; Conradi, S.; Delmotte, M.H.; Lanteri-Minet, M.; Lefaucheur, J.P.; Mick, G.; Piano, V.; et al. Pharmacological and non-pharmacological treatments for neuropathic pain: Systematic review and French recommendations. *Rev. Neurol.* **2020**, *176*, 325–352. [CrossRef] [PubMed]
42. Morra, M.E.; Elgebaly, A.; Elmaraezy, A.; Khalil, A.M.; Altibi, A.M.; Vu, T.L.; Mostafa, M.R.; Huy, N.T.; Hirayama, K. Therapeutic efficacy and safety of Botulinum Toxin A Therapy in Trigeminal Neuralgia: A systematic review and meta-analysis of randomized controlled trials. *J. Headache Pain* **2016**, *17*, 63. [CrossRef] [PubMed]

toxins

Case Report

Tardive Oromandibular Dystonia Induced by Trazodone: A Clinical Case and Management from the Perspective of the Dental Specialist

Nicolás P. Skarmeta [1,2,3], Giannina C. Katzmann [1,2], Constanza Valdés [1], Dominique Gaedechens [3] and Francisca C. Montini [1,*]

1 Facultad de Odontología, Universidad de los Andes, Santiago 7620001, Chile
2 Hospital del Salvador, Providencia 7500922, Chile
3 OPH Clinic, Vitacura 7630000, Chile
* Correspondence: fmontini@uandes.cl; Tel.: +56-2-2618-1372

Abstract: Background: Tardive Oromandibular Dystonia is an iatrogenic drug-induced movement form of extrapyramidal symptoms associated primarily with chronic consumption of dopamine receptor blocking agents. Tardive symptoms attributable to selective serotonin reuptake inhibitors antidepressants are far less prevalent. Clinical Case: The authors will present a clinical case and management, from the dental specialist perspective, of a 55-year-old female patient who developed tardive oromandibular dystonia induced by Trazodone prescribed for sleep insomnia. Conclusions: Trazodone-induced oromandibular dystonia is extremely rare. Early identification and assessment of tardive symptoms are imperative for successful treatment. Trazodone should be prescribed with caution in patients taking other medications with the potential to cause tardive syndromes.

Keywords: oromandibular dystonia; tardive dystonia; trazodone; botulinum toxin

Key Contribution: The authors present a rare case of tardive oromandibular dystonia induced by chronic consumption of Trazodone; demonstrating how the dental specialist can contribute to the early recognition; assessment; and successful treatment.

Citation: Skarmeta, N.P.; Katzmann, G.C.; Valdés, C.; Gaedechens, D.; Montini, F.C. Tardive Oromandibular Dystonia Induced by Trazodone: A Clinical Case and Management from the Perspective of the Dental Specialist. *Toxins* **2022**, *14*, 680. https://doi.org/10.3390/toxins14100680

Received: 22 August 2022
Accepted: 23 September 2022
Published: 30 September 2022

1. Introduction

Oromandibular movement disorders (OMD) are a group of hyperkinetic motor disorders which affect the muscles of mastication, the face, and the tongue. From an etiologic standpoint, these disorders may be acquired, inherited, or idiopathic [1].

Acquired OMD can be attributed to perinatal brain injuries, infections, trauma, ischemic/hemorrhagic cerebrovascular accidents, arteriovenous malformations, toxicity, and drugs [2].

Drug-induced OMD encompasses a wide variety of hyperkinetic and hypokinetic extrapyramidal involuntary movements, manifesting in the form of dystonia, tremors, stereotypy, tics, dyskinesia, or a combination of different types of abnormal movements [3]. The magnitude and complexity of these abnormal movements can vary from being almost unnoticeable to producing complete social impairment.

The onset of these iatrogenic movement disorders has been primarily associated with the consumption of dopamine receptor blocking agents (typical and atypical neuroleptics) and other medications such as antidepressants (e.g., tricyclic antidepressants, selective serotonin reuptake inhibitors, and selective norepinephrine serotonin reuptake inhibitors), antiemetics, and other medications used in gastrointestinal disorders [4].

Since the motor response to the offending drug is highly variable among patients, it is easier to categorize drug-induced OMD based on the temporal profile (i.e., the patient's exposure to the drug). Acute drug-induced OMD often occurs within hours or days after the exposure to the offending drug; in subacute drug-induced OMD, symptoms appear more slowly within days or weeks after the exposure; and tardive OMD often refers to chronic exposure to the drug, at least three months or one month in patients older than 60 years of age [3,5].

Diagnosis and recognition of these involuntary motor disorders can be elusive. In this article, the authors will present a clinical case of tardive oromandibular dystonia attributable to Trazodone prescription for sleep insomnia.

2. Clinical Case

A 55-year-old female patient was referred to the orofacial pain unit of the OPH clinic for showing symptoms of temporomandibular joint arthralgia and osteoarthritis, orofacial myofascial pain, and sleep bruxism. An experienced Orofacial Pain Specialist performed a comprehensive clinical history and examination following the Diagnostic Criteria for Temporomandibular Disorders (DC/TMD) protocol and the International Classification of Orofacial Pain-1 (ICOP-1) criteria. At the moment of the examination, the patient was taking 150 mg of Venlafaxine for major depressive disorder, 4 mg of Clonazepam for sleep onset insomnia, and hormone replacement therapy for menopause.

Another major complaint of the patient was difficulty initiating and maintaining sleep. Thus, an Epworth Sleepiness Scale and Insomnia Severity Index were performed to complete the sleep evaluation. Due to the high scores presented by the patient and clinical history consistent with chronic sleep insomnia, polysomnography (PSG) was requested Even though the PSG revealed no sleep breathing disorders, the exam showed severe modifications in the patient's sleep architecture, a mild increase in the arousal index, and low-frequency sleep bruxism. (Table 1) The PSG results led us to hypothesize that the patient's sleep architecture alterations were because of the chronic consumption of benzodiazepines. Thus, the patient was derived to her treating psychiatrist to gradually diminish and eliminate the intake of Clonazepam.

Table 1. REM sleep stages, Arousal Index, Sleep Bruxism Index.

Sleep Stages	Arousal Index	Sleep Bruxism Index
NREM1 (10.0%) NREM2 (75.9%) NREM3 (14.3%) REM (0.0%)	16.4 eps per hour	2.4 eps per hour

During this time, the patient successfully underwent her osteoarthritis and orofacial myofascial pain treatment. In addition, an upper oral occlusal splint was prescribed to manage low-frequency sleep bruxism.

In order to manage sleep initiation and maintenance insomnia, the psychiatrist tapered the dosage of Clonazepam and progressively replaced it with Trazodone until a target dose of 100 mg was reached. Throughout this period, the patient did not experience any extrapyramidal symptoms.

Almost three months later, after the end of the orofacial pain treatment, the patient returned complaining of a sudden worsening of her awake bruxism. The patient presented abrupt rhythmic involuntary muscle contractions, similar to jaw-closing and jaw-deviating dystonic-like movements affecting the right side of her masticatory muscles. (See Figure 1, and Supplemental Videos S1 and S2) The dystonic-like episodes were spontaneous or triggered by everyday activities such as talking, chewing, and yawning. The severity of these motor contractions tended to be exacerbated by emotional stress and nervousness produced by these uncontrollable movements. During these episodes, some typical features of oromandibular dystonia were noticed, such as some sensory tricks (gentle pressure on the inferior incisors would milden the jaw-deviating dystonia as the placement of a tongue depressor between the molars for jaw-closing dystonia), and phenomena (e.g., oromandibular dystonia overflowing the right eyelid, resulting in right blepharospasm).

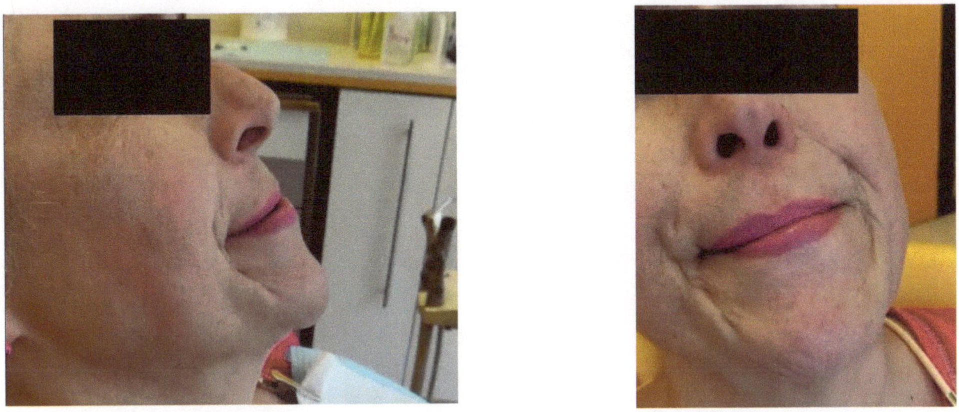

(a) (b)

Figure 1. (**a**) Jaw-deviating and closing dystonia producing episodes of forceful clothing and protrusive movements; (**b**) Jaw-deviating dystonia to the left side producing forceful contractions of the inferior head of the right lateral pterygoid muscle.

A video examination protocol suggested by Yoshida was carried out to assess the type and magnitude of involuntary movements [6]. In addition, a complete haematological and biochemical blood examination was required and all the parameters were within normal range. Thus, both thyroid and parathyroid hormonal dysfunction were ruled out.

Since the literature indicates that Trazodone can induce extrapyramidal symptoms and abnormal oromandibular movement disorders only start after the addition of this medication. The authors, in agreement with her treating physician, suggested performing a slow taper until complete discontinuation of Trazodone was achieved.

A progressive dose reduction of 25 mg of Trazodone was scheduled every two weeks. In the meantime, an inferior occlusal splint was prescribed, considering that mild contact in the inferior incisor tended to ease the intensity of the dystonic-like movements.

During the progressive discontinuation of Trazodone, the authors noticed an immediate attenuation of the dystonic symptoms. However, only achieving a partial but clear remission of them. No video protocol was recorded during the tampering of Trazodone.

Considering that the patient's mental health status was stable, it was decided to take a more conservative approach, only eliminating the most likely offending drug, namely, Trazodone. Consequently, the authors maintained that Venlafaxine intake was unchanged in order not to jeopardize the psychiatric treatment, and also closely monitored the evolution of the clinical symptoms. Additionally, the authors indicated the administration of 25 units of incobotulium toxin (Xeomin®, Merz, Germany) per masseter muscle, 20 units per temporalis muscle, and 15 units were applied to the inferior head of the right lateral pterygoid with electrical stimulation guidance (See anatomical landmarks in Figure 2).

During the two-week follow-up consultation, the authors could recognize a substantial decrease in the magnitude and intensity of the oromandibular movement. Two months and seven months after the discontinuation of the offending drug and botulinum toxin application, the authors re-recorded Yoshida's video protocol to carry out an objective before and after comparison of the treatment results. See Table 2 for comparison prior to and after the treatment.

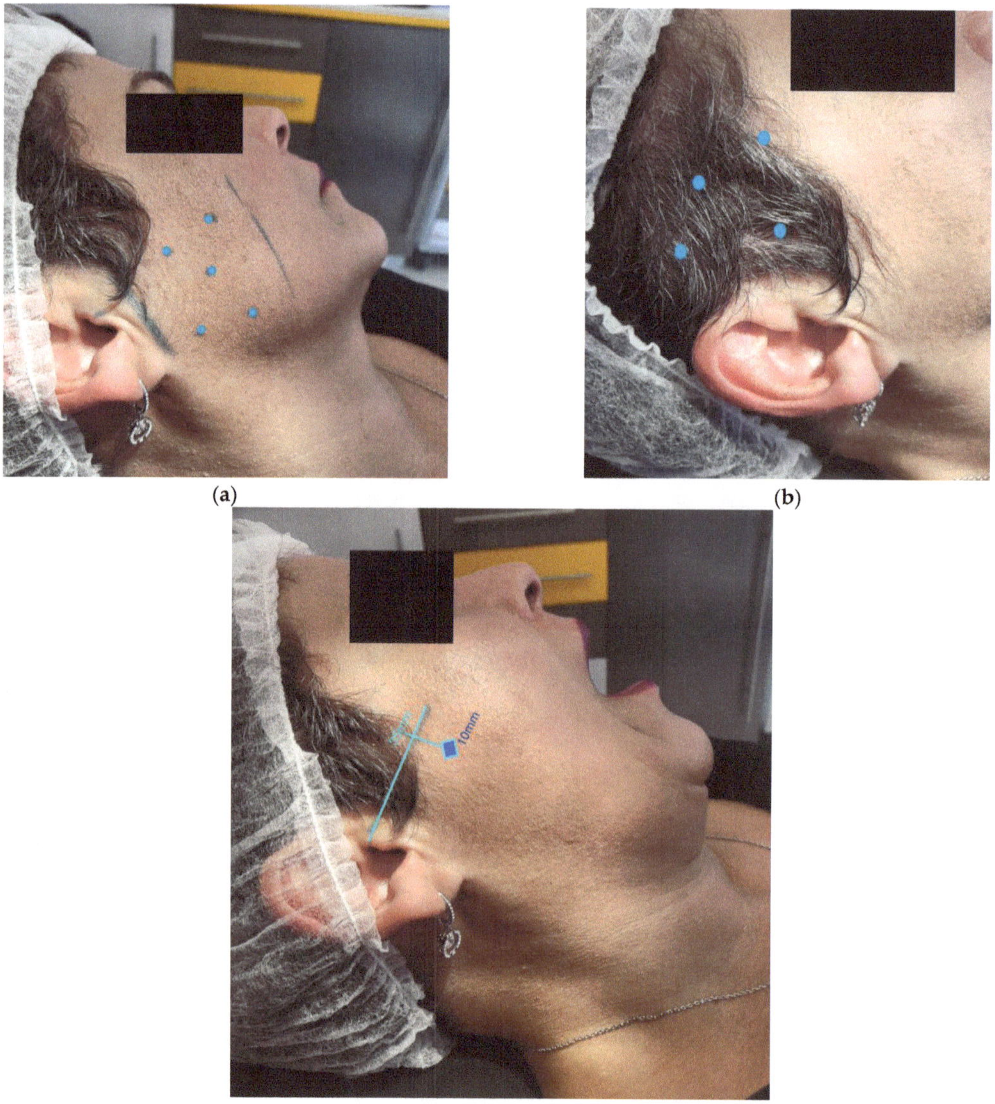

(a) (b) (c)

Figure 2. (**a**) Incobotulinum toxin injection sites for the masseter muscle; (**b**) Incobotulinum toxin injection sites for the temporalis muscle. (**c**) Anatomic landmarks for extraoral injection with electrical stimulation guidance to the inferior head of the right lateral pterygoid muscle.

Table 2. Yoshida's Video examination Protocol for OMD.

Examination Protocol for OMD	Prior Treatment *	Two-Month Follow-Up *	Seven-Month Follow-Up *
At rest (10 s)	4	0	0
Counting 1 to 10 out loud	2	0	0
Open/Close mouth (5 times)	2	0	0

Table 2. *Cont.*

Examination Protocol for OMD	Prior Treatment *	Two-Month Follow-Up *	Seven-Month Follow-Up *
Lateral Movements (5 times)	3	0	0
Jaw Protrusion (5 times)	5	0	0
Tongue Protrusion (hold for 5 s)	0	0	0
Hold a long vowel (5–10 s)	0	0	0
Read a Sentence	2	0	0
Gum chewing (30 s)	4	0	0

* Number of involuntary dystonic episodes triggered by different mandibular activities.

3. Discussion

Antidepressant Drug-induced extrapyramidal symptoms are considered a rare cluster of severe adverse reactions which cause considerable morbidity and significantly impair the quality of life [7].

Tardive syndromes are usually produced by chronic exposure to dopamine receptor blocking agents (DRBA), such as typical and atypical antipsychotics. However, other medications such as tricyclic antidepressants (TCAs), serotonin reuptake inhibitors antidepressants (SSRIs), and medications used for gastrointestinal disorders can also produce extrapyramidal symptoms [3,4].

The plausible mechanisms involved in iatrogenic drug-induced movements disorders are usually related to a drug-induced extended occupancy of dopamine D2 receptors, which may be related to a hypothetical post-synaptic supersensitivity and upregulation of dopamine receptors, resulting in the disinhibition of the globulus pallidum internus and the subthalamic nucleus, which, in turn, can produce a wide variety of hyperkinetic manifestations [3].

In particular, the theoretical link between SSRIs and the onset of tardive syndromes may be related to the antagonism of 5HT2 receptors in the GABA-ergic interneurons of the nigrostriatal pathway, which can lead to the suppression of the activity of these dopaminergic neurons explaining the occurrence of hyperkinetic movement disorders. The incidence of extrapyramidal movement disorders with these pharmacological compounds is relatively low. In fact, the estimated risk of developing these disorders is lower than 1 in 1000 [8].

Trazodone is a triazolopyridine derivative from the serotonin 5HT2A and 5HT2c receptor antagonist and belongs to the reuptake inhibitors class of antidepressants, approved for major depressive disorder. Additionally, it is commonly used as an off-label medication to treat delirium and insomnia, because it displays a moderately potent antagonist effect over alpha 1A and 2A adrenoreceptors and H1 histaminergic receptors, which is probably related to its sedative effect [9,10].

Another plausible mechanism that may explain how Trazodone may trigger extrapyramidal symptoms is its inhibitory effect on T-type calcium channels, exerting a similar effect in the subthalamic nucleus similar to other medications related to tardive syndromes such as haloperidol and flunarizine [11,12].

To the authors' knowledge, there is scarce literature reporting trazodone-induced tardive symptoms. Furthermore, the authors only found a few reports of tardive dystonic symptoms after chronic consumption of Trazadone [12,13].

Treatment recommendations in tardive syndromes often start with progressive tampering with the offending drug. In fact, the sooner the causative drug is removed, the likelier the tardive symptoms will be solved.

Pharmacological management often varies depending on the severity of the symptoms, the type of drug inducing the symptoms (i.e., DRBAs, TCAs, SSRIs), and the chronicity of intake.

The most common therapeutic approach suggested in the literature, besides a progressive taper of the offending drug, is the use of Dopamine-depleting agents such as Tetrabenazine and Reserpine; Antiparkinson agents such as Amantadine; GABA agonists such as Clonazepam, Valproic Acid, and Baclofen; Anticholinergic agents such as Trihexyphenidyl, and Chemodenervation with botulinum toxin [3].

In this clinical case, the oromandibular movement disorders were consistent with tardive dystonia. Consequently, the authors chose the abovementioned treatment strategy based on the phenomenology of tardive symptoms. In this clinical case, we performed chemodenervation using botulinum toxin in the dystonic masticatory muscles [14], installed a diurnal inferior oral appliance (to produce a sensory trick and protect the oral structures) [15], and carried out a progressive reduction and removal of the offending drug. The treatment successfully achieved a complete attenuation of the abnormal movement disorders.

4. Conclusions

Tardive syndromes may severely affect the quality of life and produce substantial social impairment. Hence, treating tardive symptoms is complex, especially because sometimes symptoms may be treated successfully. Thus, preventing and identifying the onset of tardive syndromes is of paramount importance. Although the risk of producing tardive syndrome induced by Trazodone is extremely low, clinicians should balance the risk/benefit ratio before prescribing drugs that can potentially produce tardive symptoms. Moreover, prescribing Trazodone for insomnia or delirium should be avoided completely or done only when it is strictly necessary for patients with the chronic intake of other drugs with the potential to induce tardive syndromes. The authors' recommendation to health professionals, based on this unusual clinical case, is to avoid drug-on-drug interactions whenever possible and prefer medications that have less potential of producing tardive syndromes.

Supplementary Materials: The following supporting information can be downloaded at: https://www.mdpi.com/article/10.3390/toxins14100680/s1, Video S1: Tardive Dystonia from a Sagital Plane; Video S2: Tardive Dystonia from a frontal plane.

Author Contributions: N.P.S. acted as the main clinician, documented the case, and contributed in the conceptualization and writing the original draft. G.C.K. contributed in the original draft preparation and editing. C.V. contributed in the original draft preparation and editing. D.G. contributed documenting the case and reviewing and editing the draft. F.C.M. contributed in writing the original draft and reviewing and editing the manuscript. All authors have read and agreed to the published version of the manuscript.

Funding: This research received no external funding.

Institutional Review Board Statement: Not applicable.

Informed Consent Statement: Written informed consent has been obtained from the patient to publish this paper.

Data Availability Statement: Not applicable.

Conflicts of Interest: The authors declare no conflict of interest.

References

1. Grütz, K.; Klein, C. Dystonia updates: Definition, nomenclature, clinical classification, and etiology. *J. Neural. Transm.* **2021**, *128*, 395–404. [CrossRef] [PubMed]
2. Albanese, A.; Bhatia, K.; Bressman, S.B.; DeLong, M.R.; Fahn, S.; Fung, V.S.; Hallett, M.; Jankovic, J.; Jinnah, H.A.; Klein, C.; et al. Phenomenology and classification of dystonia: A consensus update. *Mov. Disord.* **2013**, *28*, 863–873. [CrossRef] [PubMed]
3. Waln, O.; Jankovic, J. An update on tardive dyskinesia: From phenomenology to treatment. *Tremor Other Hyperkinet. Mov.* **2013**, *3*, 1–11. [CrossRef] [PubMed]
4. Savitt, D.; Jankovic, J. Tardive syndromes. *J. Neurol. Sci.* **2018**, *389*, 35–42. [CrossRef] [PubMed]

5. Skármeta, N.P.; Espinoza-Mellado, P.; Chana, P. Orofacial dystonia and other oromandibular movement disorders. In *Dystonia-Different Prospects*; Rizk, T.M.G., Ed.; IntechOpen: London, UK, 2018; Available online: https://www.intechopen.com/chapters/62475 (accessed on 31 August 2022). [CrossRef]
6. Yoshida, K. Development and Validation of a Disease-Specific Oromandibular Dystonia Rating Scale (OMDRS). *Front. Neurol.* **2020**, *11*, 583177. [CrossRef] [PubMed]
7. Madhusoodanan, S.; Alexeenko, L.; Sanders, R.; Brenner, R. Extrapyramidal symptoms associated with antidepressants—A review of the literature and an analysis of spontaneous reports. *Ann. Clin. Psychiatry* **2010**, *22*, 148–156. [PubMed]
8. Guo, M.Y.; Etminan, M.; Procyshyn, R.M.; Kim, D.D.; Samii, A.; Kezouh, A.; Carleton, B.C. Association of Antidepressant Use with Drug-Related Extrapyramidal Symptoms: A Pharmacoepidemiological Study. *J. Clin. Psychopharmacol.* **2018**, *38*, 349–356. [CrossRef] [PubMed]
9. Brogden, R.N.; Heel, R.C.; Speight, T.M.; Avery, G.S. Trazodone: A Review of its Pharmacological Properties and Therapeutic Use in Depression and Anxiety. *Drugs* **1981**, *21*, 401–429. [CrossRef] [PubMed]
10. Cuomo, A.; Bianchetti, A.; Cagnin, A.; De Berardis, D.; Di Fazio, I.; Incalzi, R.A.; Marra, C.; Neviani, F.; Laurenzi, P.F.; Nicoletti, F. Trazodone: A multifunctional antidepressant. Evaluation of its properties and real-world use. *J. Gerontol. Geriatr.* **2021**, *69*, 120–129. [CrossRef]
11. Kraus, R.L.; Li, Y.; Jovanovska, A.; Renger, J.J. Trazodone inhibits T-type calcium channels. *Neuropharmacology* **2007**, *53*, 308–317. [CrossRef] [PubMed]
12. Kadota, Y.; Hori, H.; Takayama, M.; Okabe, C.; Ohara, N. Tardive dystonia improved with discontinuation of trazodone in an elderly schizophrenia patient: A case report. *Ann. Gen. Psychiatry* **2020**, *19*, 23. [CrossRef] [PubMed]
13. Lin, C.C.; Lin, P.Y.; Chang, Y.Y.; Chen, C.H.; Lee, Y. Tardive dystonia and tardive sensory syndrome related to trazodone: A case report. *Prog. Neuro-Psychopharmacol. Biol. Psychiatry* **2008**, *32*, 1609–1610. [CrossRef] [PubMed]
14. Yoshida, K. Botulinum Toxin Therapy for Oromandibular Dystonia and Other Movement Disorders in the Stomatognathic System. *Toxins* **2022**, *14*, 282. [CrossRef] [PubMed]
15. Yoshida, K. Sensory trick splint as a multimodal therapy for oromandibular dystonia. *J. Prosthodont. Res.* **2018**, *62*, 239–244. [CrossRef] [PubMed]

MDPI AG
Grosspeteranlage 5
4052 Basel
Switzerland
Tel.: +41 61 683 77 34

Toxins Editorial Office
E-mail: toxins@mdpi.com
www.mdpi.com/journal/toxins

www.ingramcontent.com/pod-product-compliance
Lightning Source LLC
Chambersburg PA
CBHW042010260926
51850CB00020B/2948
9783725820931